Contents

Introduction

Many people love herbs. They enjoy their colour, taste and scent. They may feel confident to add several to their meals but they're not at all sure about using herbs to make other things such as infused oils or tinctures. The aim of this book is to develop confidence; to be able to take a herbal harvest and create a variety of useful items which will help support individuals, families and the local community.

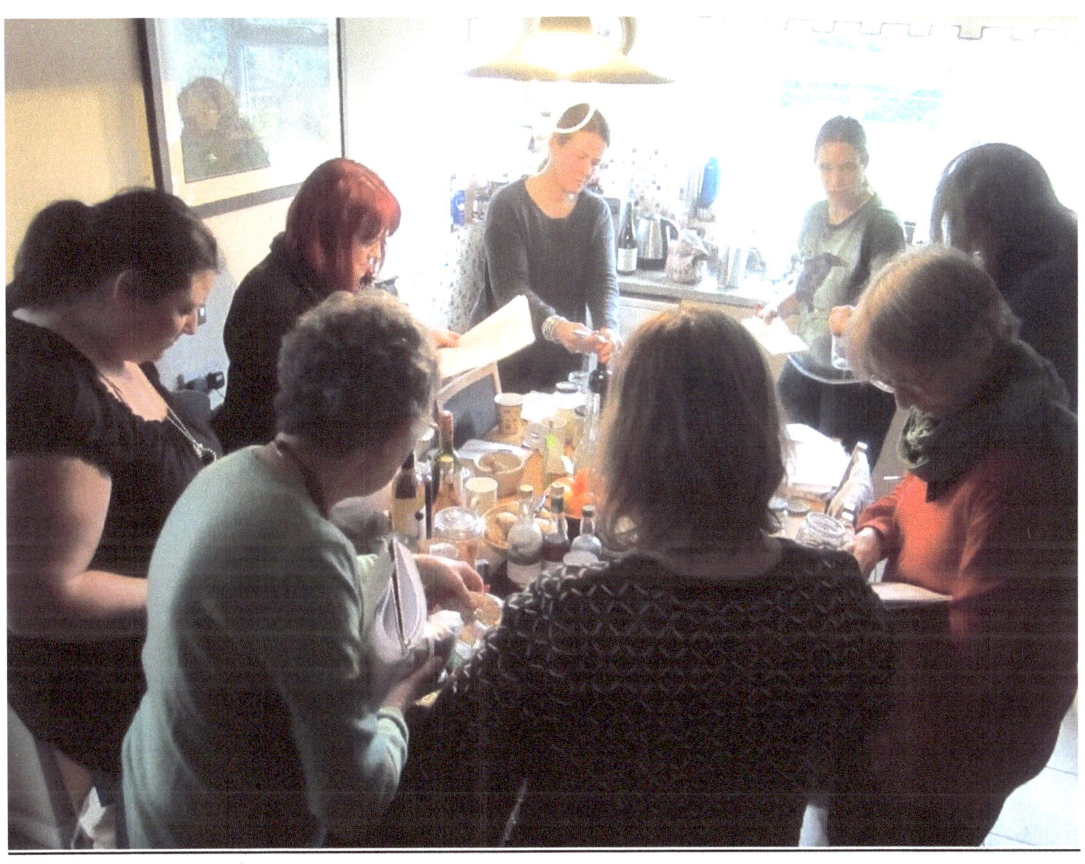

Playing with herbs in the kitchen

Herbal terminology

In every craft, there are words which are used to mean specific things. Playing with herbs is no different. Here are a few of the most commonly used terms with a brief explanation of what they mean.

Cream – product made for external application onto skin by vigorously combining salve (oil) with a liquid (tincture or tea).

Cold water maceration – this is where cold water is poured over plant material in a bowl and left overnight in a cool place. The liquid is strained and used the next morning.

Cordial – a liquid made from a sweetened herbal tea and diluted before drinking with hot or cold water.

Decoction – the method of extracting active plant elements by heating in a covered saucepan, bringing to the boil and simmering for 15-30 minutes.

Electuary – powdered herbs mixed into honey or jam and eaten.

Elixir – herbal extraction with equal quantities of brandy and honey.

Essential oil - extremely concentrated, fragrant oil produced by distilling plant matter. (Cannot be made at home without a still.)

Extraction – the means by which you remove the active ingredients from a herb.

Febrifuge - medicine used to reduce fever

Flower essence – the process of extracting the energetic essence of a flower into water and preserved with alcohol. Often used for emotional maladies.

Fomentation – where a clean piece of cloth is dipped in a strong, hot herbal tea and applied to area of need. Good for cramps, bruises, aches etc.

Herbal oil – an infused oil produced by heating plant material in the sun for a period of time (single sun infusion), or by dividing an amount of herb in half and heating each half in the same amount of base oil for two hours in a water bath with external heat source (double infusion).

Honey – aromatic herbs infused in honey.

Honey pills – powdered herbs mixed with honey and dried.

'Knit-bone' – a herb which stimulates the growth of new cells following bone fracture

Long hot infusion – where boiling water (usually 1 litre/2 UK pints) is poured over an amount of herb (usually 50g/2ozs dried) and left to infuse overnight. The liquid is then strained and drunk either cold or hot.

Maceration – a method of extracting water-soluble elements of a herb by means of a cold liquid e.g. water, alcohol or vinegar. The timing will be different depending on the menstrum. Water is usually overnight, alcohol and vinegar three weeks, cold oil six weeks, honey four to six weeks, honey and brandy four to six weeks.

Marc – the plant matter placed in a menstrum whilst making a tincture.

Menstrum – the medium used to extract active plant elements e.g. alcohol.

Oxymel – hot drink made from mixing 2 tsps. infused cider vinegar with 2 tsps. honey/infused herbal honey in a mug of boiling water (a mint or rose or elderflower oxymel can be made with iced water for a cooling summer drink)

Poultice – chopped herb moistened with hot water or oil, placed in a bandage and applied to the skin.

Salve – product made for external application onto skin by heating beeswax with an infused herbal oil which will solidify on cooling.

Spit poultice – made by chewing a leaf or flower head until thoroughly mashed, then applied to skin and fixed with bandage.

Suppositories – herbal powders mixed with cocoa butter and inserted anally or vaginally.

Syrup – a liquid sweetened with sugar or honey made from a concentrated/reduced herbal tea with sugar or honey added in the concentration of 1Kg/1lb per 1litre/20 fluid oz. of tea. Usually taken by the spoonful.

Tea – this is a liquid made by pouring just boiled water over an amount of fresh or dried plant material and leaving it to infuse for ten minutes. Teas can be drunk, made into syrups or cordials, used in a poultice or fomentation or poured over sickly plants when cold.

Tincture – Herbal properties extracted in alcohol

Vinegar – herbal properties and minerals extracted in vinegar, usually cider vinegar.

Notes

Chapter One

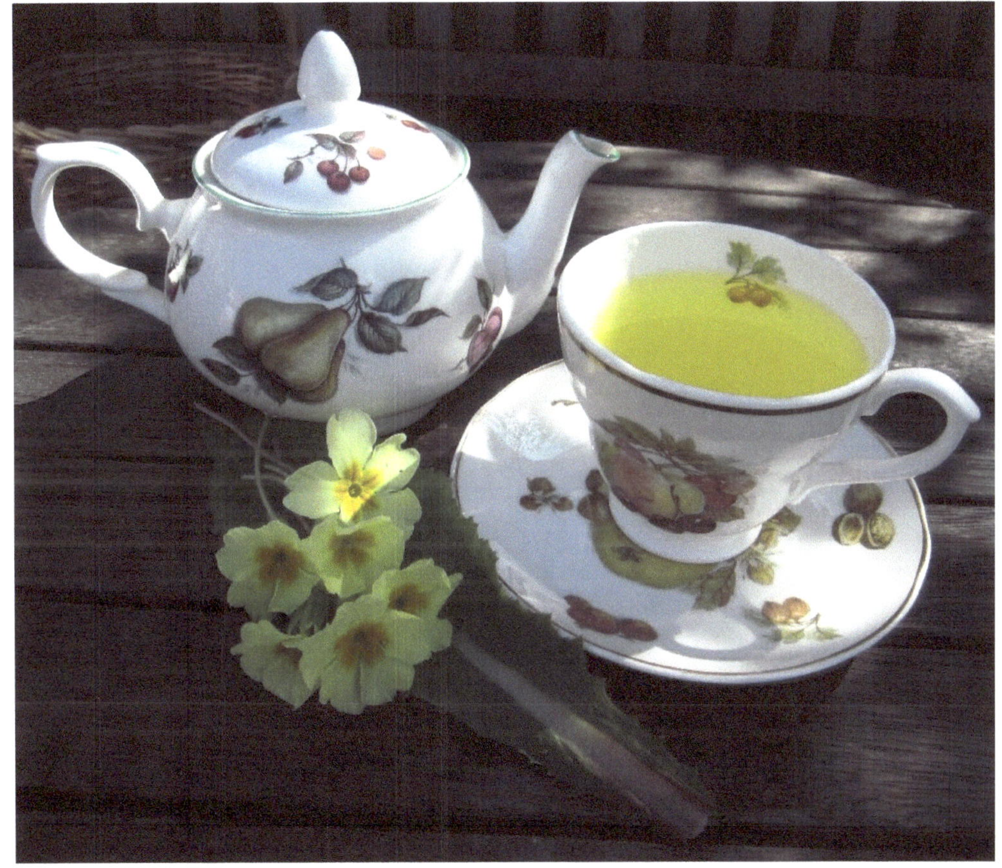

Primrose tea

Using hot and cold water

Infusions

(i)   Tea

An infusion is often called a tea. They are not produced instantly. The aim is to pour "just-boiled" water onto fresh or dried leaf, flower or stem of a plant to infuse the water-soluble components so you can drink the resulting liquid. You don't want the water to be boiling at one hundred degrees centigrade when you pour it on, or a lot of the aromatic oils will disappear in the steam. You can avoid this by placing the herb in a glass or ceramic (not metal) teapot or cafetiere (French press). Anything with a lid will do. If you have one of the large tea mugs with a lid they use in the Orient, that's fine too.

The amount of herb used depends on whether you have fresh or dried. Fresh herbs contain a greater amount of water, so usually one tablespoon of fresh herb equals one teaspoon of dried herb.

Teas can be "simples" which means they are made from one herb, or "combinations".

The usual amount for one cup of herb tea is 2 tsp herb to one cup of boiling water. Leave the herb to steep for 10 minutes and then drink. Most herbs have a dosage that says drink one cup of herb tea three times a day. You can make a pint's worth (500ml) and store it in the fridge and heat up your 1/3 pint as and when you need it. However, it is part of the healing process to spend time making the tea, so it is often preferable to make each cup of tea with fresh ingredients.

I have an aversion to measuring. My usual method of making tea is to add two pinches of dried herb or a small handful of fresh herb into a small, one-person cafetiere and fill it to the top with just boiled water. I depress the plunger after ten minutes then pour the herb tea into a mug. Depending on the size of my mug, there may be some left to drink later.

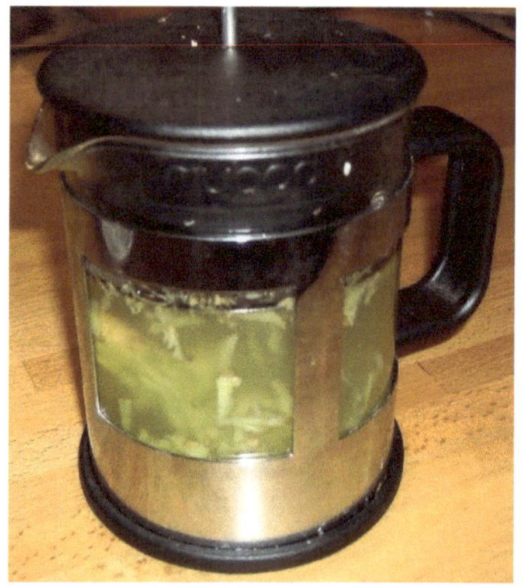

Ginger tea brewing in a cafatiere

<u>Recipes for pleasant teas</u>

Several herbs taste good on their own. Try lemon balm, lime flower, cleavers, ground elder, young nettles, catmint, chocolate or red mint for easily accessible, refreshing teas.

Nettle Latte - Make a strong infusion of dried or young, fresh nettles together with half a cinnamon stick or 1tsp. powdered cinnamon plus grated nutmeg and one clove. You can also add grated ginger root for added warmth. Heat a portion of milk and whisk until frothy. Mix hot milk and hot nettle tea in equal quantities. Add honey to taste. This tea is equally delicious with or without the milk. You can add almond milk if you prefer.

<u>Anti-viral/cough combinations</u>

Cold tea – equal quantities of peppermint, yarrow and elderflower

Post-viral tea – 1tsp each of dried sage and thyme with 1inch of grated or chopped root ginger infused for ten minutes then poured over the juice of half a lemon with honey to taste.

Calendula tea – infuse 1tsp of dried calendula petals with water.

Other anti-viral/anti-bacterial herbs include bergamot and New England aster. Bergamot (both the red and purple varieties) can be very strong so use sparingly.

<u>Soothing teas</u>

Bedtime tea - lemon balm, lime flower and chamomile.

IDGAS tea – vervain, lemon balm and chamomile (Use when stressed. Can be helpful in terminal care for both patient and family)

<u>Cooling teas</u>

Elderflower and sage can both be used as simples for hot flushes

Boneset and elderflower can be used as febrifuges to break and bring down fevers in both children and adults. (Boneset is very bitter!)

> (ii)   Long infusions

Some mineral-rich herbs can benefit from overnight infusions. These can be made in a thermos flask or your usual container. They are often made in larger quantities than a simple tea and in combinations to give a pleasant taste by adding aromatic herbs to the mix.

To make a long infusion add equal parts of fresh or dried herbs to produce around 2oz/50g dried or 8oz/200g fresh herbs. Pour over 2pints/1litre boiling water, cover and leave overnight. In the morning, strain and decant into another container and keep in the fridge to drink throughout the day.

Herbs used in long infusions are nettle, violet, red clover, oatstraw. Mint, hibiscus, lemon balm, lemon verbena or other pleasantly flavoured herbs can be added if desired.

> (iii)   Using Teas externally

> a) <u>Eyes</u>

Eyebright is the most effective herb for any eye condition. If you have runny eyes with your cold, try making eyebright tea. Use a portion in an eye bath and drink the remainder. You could also make a compress by soaking a clean piece of cloth or kitchen towel in the cooled tea and applying it to your eyes.

Other useful eye herbs are: -

- Eyebright and cleavers -for infections
- Eyebright, calendula, chamomile, elderflower and rose – for conjunctivitis
- Chamomile, nettle, lemon balm, yarrow, feverfew and Baikal skullcap – for allergic reactions
- Goldenrod – for hay fever and cat allergies
- Cleavers – when you get grit in your eyes
- Elderflower, chamomile, calendula, plantain and roses – for tired or strained eyes (especially from computer usage)
- Eyebright and goldenrod – for dry eyes when the kidneys are implicated

b) Pain

For any kind of smooth muscle pain, soak a piece of clean cloth in a strong tea and apply to the aching area. This is known as using a fomentation or compress and allows the herb to pass through the skin to relax the constricted internal muscle. It is useful for period pains, IBS pain, pulled muscles and other similar conditions where warmth can be comforting.

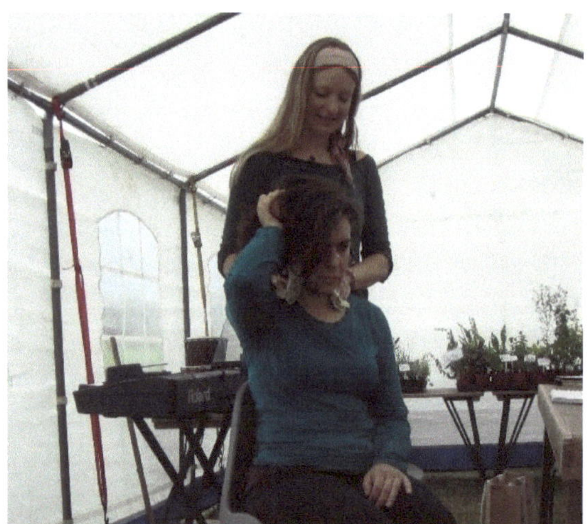

Herbalist Lucinda Warner applying a fomentation to soothe aching neck muscles on Springfield Sanctuary apprentice, Nuria, in 2011.

The principle herb used in fomentations is chamomile. You can also use fomentations when cooling is called for, e.g. in inflammatory conditions such as arthritis.

The principle herbs for cooling are yarrow, plantain and elderflower.

c) Bath herbs

Adding herbal tea to bath water is an ancient and easy way to administer herbs. The active components are absorbed through the skin. This is an ideal way to soothe over-tired and fractious children.

Children's bath combination – lavender, lemon balm and chamomile

If there is no time or ability to relax in a bath, try a hand or foot soak for fifteen minutes.

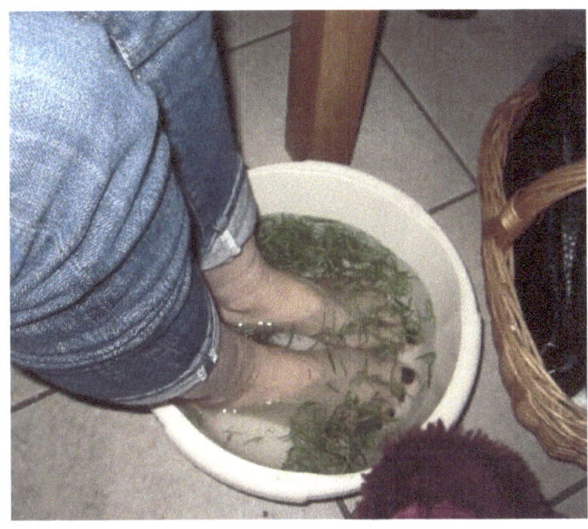

- For circulatory problems – ginger

- For diabetic neuropathy – St John's wort flowers

- General soothing – rosemary, elderflower and lavender

A sitz or hip bath can also be used for administering herbs especially after childbirth.

Decoction

A decoction is a tea made with stems, dried seeds or roots and boiled gently in a saucepan for 10-20 minutes. You use this with any material that needs to "break down" a little to release the aromatic oils. Don't use an aluminium saucepan. Use 1oz/25g of herb to 1 pint/500ml of water. Remember to put the lid on the saucepan so that you don't lose too much of the liquid.

Examples of herbs to be decocted would be burdock root, hawthorn berries, dandelion root. If you are making a combination of leaves and roots/stems, make the decoction first with the roots and seeds then strain the liquid onto the leaves and allow the herbs to infuse for ten minutes.

Decoctions can be kept in the fridge for up to three days.

Warming winter tea

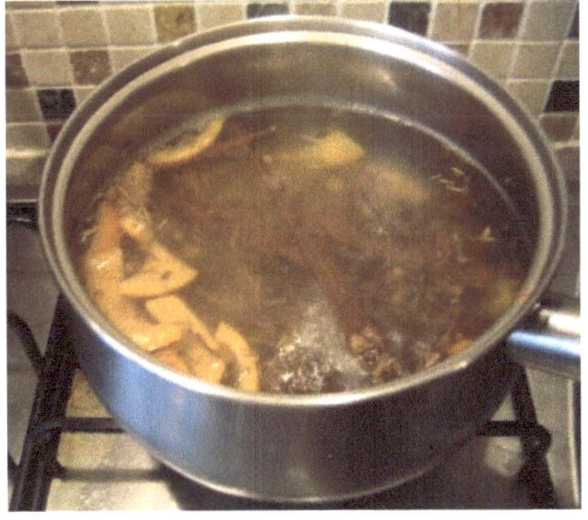

Place 1-2 tsp flax seed together with a broken up cinnamon stick and maybe a couple of cardamom pods and some sliced orange peel, a handful of fresh or half a handful of dried rosehips and the juice of half an orange. Put all the ingredients in a small saucepan and fill the saucepan with cold water. Bring to the boil, then simmer uncovered until the amount of water has halved from evaporation. Strain, add honey to taste and sip while hot.

Maceration

Some roots and other herbs respond better to a cold maceration rather than a decoction. Chop up about 1 oz/25g of root herb e.g. marshmallow or ashwagandha root, place in a jug or basin and pour 1 pint/500ml of cold water over the root. Leave in a cool place overnight. Next day, strain the mixture through a sieve and divide into three equal portions to drink during the day.

You can also use the maceration process to release minerals from herbs. You can release calcium from nettles by macerating them in cold water for 4 hours or overnight. Use a similar process for oat straw. Both these plants are nourishing to the body and will help with bone density loss after menopause and increase female libido and male fertility.

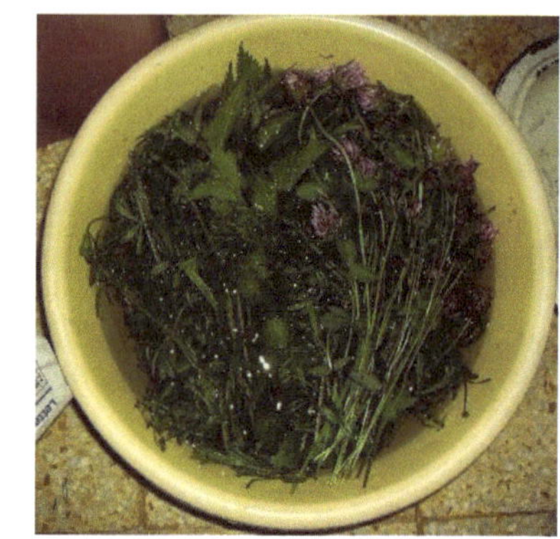

Nettle/red clover overnight maceration

Syrups and Cordials

Syrups used to be the preferred method of administering herbs to children or when a herb was particularly unpalatable. The aim was to make a strong decoction then reduce the liquid by 7/8ths of its volume by slow evaporation then add twice the weight of sugar. The extreme sugar content ensured the syrup would have a longer shelf life as both syrups and cordials are notorious for going mouldy even when kept at low temperatures in a fridge.

My preferred method is to add equal amounts of sugar to reduced liquid and I have found most syrups poured into sterile containers will last unopened for nearly a year or more. I don't reduce cordials so much and store these in small bottles in the freezer.

I use the general syrup recipe developed by London herbalists, Non Shaw and Christopher Hedley.

General syrup recipe
1 l (2 pints) water
40 g (1 1/2 oz) dried herb or 100g (4oz) fresh chopped herb
450 g (1 lb) sugar
Put herb in water, bring to a boil, let simmer 20-30 minutes, strain.
Clean out pan, pour liquid back into it, let sit on minimum heat until you only have 2 dl (7 fl.oz) left. Add sugar, simmer until sugar has dissolved, pour into jars, label. (This takes time. 1 fluid ounce evaporates about every hour.) If making a syrup with more liquid, the general rule of thumb is to add 1lb sugar or honey to every 1 pint of liquid.

A children's cough syrup can be made from onions or elderberry and echinacea in equal parts. Another cough syrup which is a delightful exercise to make with both children and adults is violet, which can also be used for constipation in children.

Violet flower Syrup

Fill a clean glass jar with violet flowers, cover with boiling water and leave overnight with

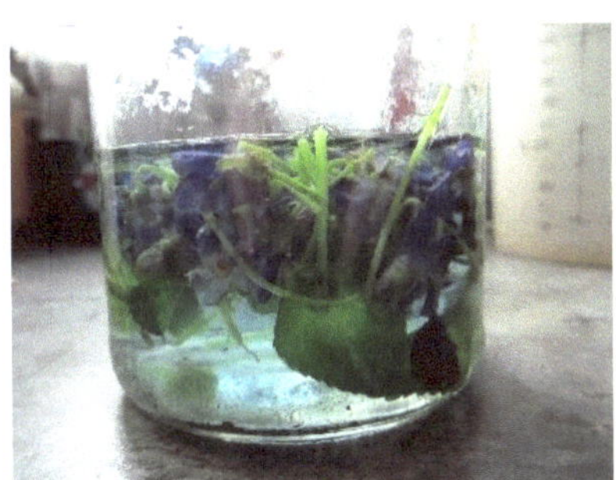

the lid screwed on. The next day, strain and measure the infused liquid. Don't worry if it looks and smells strange. For every 7fl ozs of liquid add 5 ozs of sugar. Add the juice of at least half a lemon. The liquid will turn the most delightful shade of pink! Put all the ingredients into a pan and bring to the boil and simmer for a couple of minutes. Pour the resulting syrup into a sterilized bottle or jar, seal, label and date.

Violet flower and leaf infusion

Store in the fridge and discard if it starts going mouldy. The suggested dosage for a child's cough or slight constipation is 1-2 tsps given at bedtime. If you are making this for a child under two years old and usually make your syrups with honey, use sugar this time.

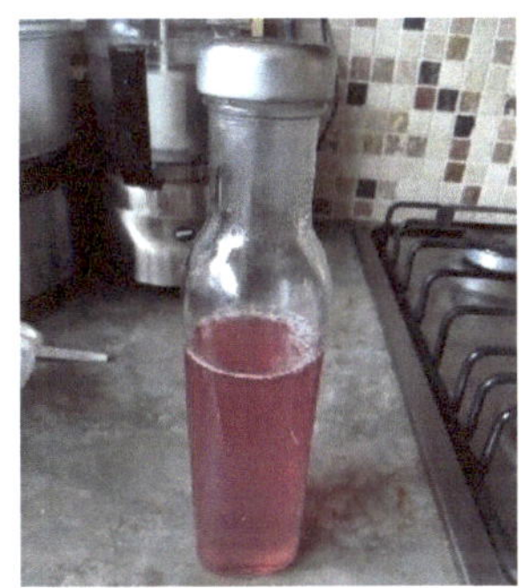

Violet syrup

Elderberry Rob

Take a quantity of elderberries and strip them from their stalks with a fork. Press out the juice using a wine press or jelly bag. I usually put them into a large piece of clean used cotton sheet and twist one end around until you can't squeeze out any more. This is a very tactile experience and you shouldn't use or wear anything you don't mind getting stained purple from the juice! Add 1tsp allspice and 1/2 tsp ginger (optional) per 2 pints of liquid in a heavy bottomed pan" (preferably stainless steel or glass) Reduce over a low heat until the juice is the consistency of molasses. Bottle and store in a cool place. Dose: Take 1tsp in a cup of hot water daily. This recipe doesn't use any sugar or honey and therefore is suitable for people with diabetes or those who don't wish to use sugar.

Blackberry and Rosehip Syrup

Small bowl of blackberries and rosehips
1 inch of fresh ginger root peeled and chopped (or you could grate it whole)
3/4 nutmeg grated
1 cinnamon stick broken up
4 cloves
Runny honey
Juice of a lemon
Alcohol of your choice (brandy, sherry, a good whisky, vodka) optional

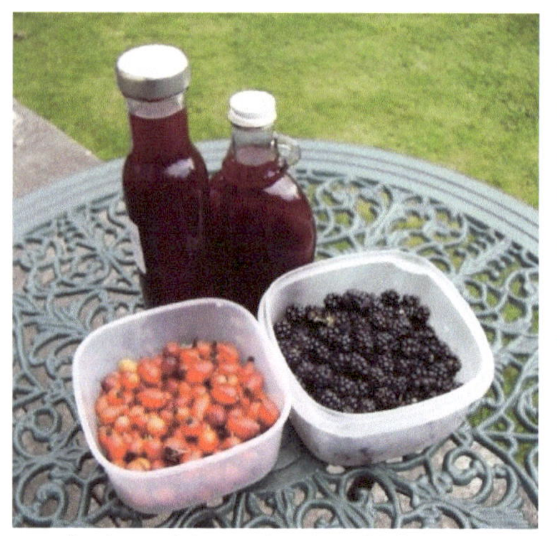

Wash the blackberries and rosehips (depending on the degree of aerial pollution). Place in a heavy-bottomed saucepan and cover with water. Simmer over a low heat for half an hour. Mash the blackberries and rosehips to a pulp with a potato masher and cook on the lowest heat for another 15-30 minutes. Strain the liquid through a plastic sieve and measure the volume. Wash out the saucepan. Return the liquid to the pan together with a lb of runny honey for every pint of liquid. Heat gently until honey is dissolved. Add juice of a lemon. This can now be poured into clean, sterile bottles and sealed and kept in the fridge to use with children and anyone who doesn't like/can't have alcohol. To preserve the syrup without keeping in fridge (but in a cold place) add alcohol to taste. I had a pint of liquid originally to which I added a pound of honey which gave around two pints of syrup so I poured out one jar then added about half a pint of Madeira to the remaining syrup. I probably could have added less. Both taste wonderful!

Blackberry cordial

1 lb blackberries
1 oz cinnamon (in sticks or powdered)
1 oz cloves (whole or powdered)
1 inch root ginger (grated)
1 lb honey/sugar
¼ pint alcohol (optional)
Cover blackberries with smallest amount of water. Add prepared spices and simmer for 20 minutes. Mash blackberries, strain and measure liquid (should be around 1 pint). Clean saucepan, pour liquid back into saucepan together with 1lb honey or sugar per pint of liquid. Heat gently, stirring until honey is dissolved. Add ¼ pint of alcohol of choice. Pour into hot, sterile bottles, seal. Label and date.

Spiced Hedgerow Cordial

1-2 lbs of blackberries
1/2lb rosehips
1 large orange (sliced)
1 and a half inches of root ginger (grated)
1 nutmeg (grated)
2 large quills of cinnamon
6 cloves
3 lbs honey
Place everything in a large pan and cover with cold water (I used about 5 pints). Bring to the boil and simmer with the lid on for about an hour. Strain the

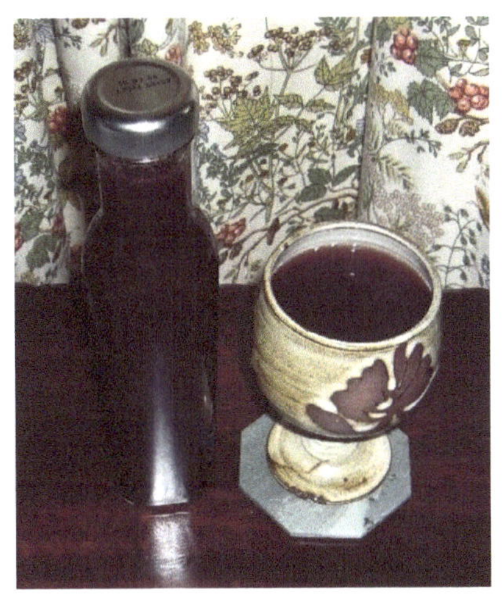

liquid and push any juicy bits you can through the sieve. Discard the debris and wash the saucepan. Measure the liquid and put on a low heat to evaporate for an hour or so, depending on how thick you want your cordial to be. A film will form on the top of the liquid, mix this back into the cordial before you add the honey. Heat very gently until the honey is dissolved. Sterilise bottles in the oven for ten minutes, then pour cordial into bottles, seal, label and date. To make the drink, add 1 tablespoon of cordial to a small cup/goblet of boiling water. Sip and enjoy.

You could use half elderberries and half blackberries and more rosehips.

Nettle Rose Syrup

Gather a large amount of fresh nettle tops and wash well. Either place in a saucepan, cover with cold water, bring to the boil, cover and simmer for twenty minutes then turn the heat off and leave overnight or place the nettles in a bowl, cover with cold water and leave overnight in a cool place. The next morning, strain the nettles and add the petals of seven red roses to the liquid in a saucepan. Bring to the boil and simmer for five minutes. Strain and measure the volume of remaining liquid. For each pint of liquid add 1lb of sugar. Stir with a wooden spoon, bring back to the boil and simmer until the syrup is reduced to

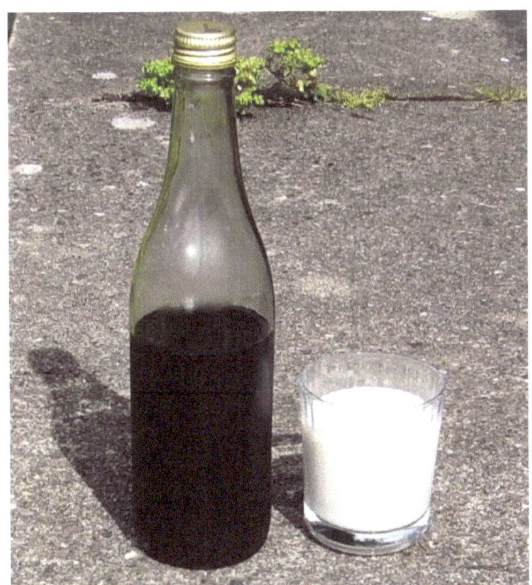

the desired consistency. Pour into heated, sterilised bottles. Seal, label and date. Store in a cool place. Keep refrigerated once opened. Use to make a milkshake with cold milk.

If you are using fresh nettles and roses together, you will need to prepare in May by cutting back an identified nettle patch to produce fresh growth in June/July when your red or pink deeply scented roses start to bloom. Otherwise use dried nettle leaves and rose petals.

If you want to maximize the mineral content of your syrup, macerate nettles in cold water overnight maybe adding red clover and/or sweet violet leaves or heartsease aerial parts. If you're looking for a soothing cough remedy, try adding marshmallow leaves to the maceration. If you want to enhance the nervine/spirit lifting effect of the roses, add Ashwagandha roots to the maceration. (Basically, the possibilities are endless!)

Rose and lemon balm cordial

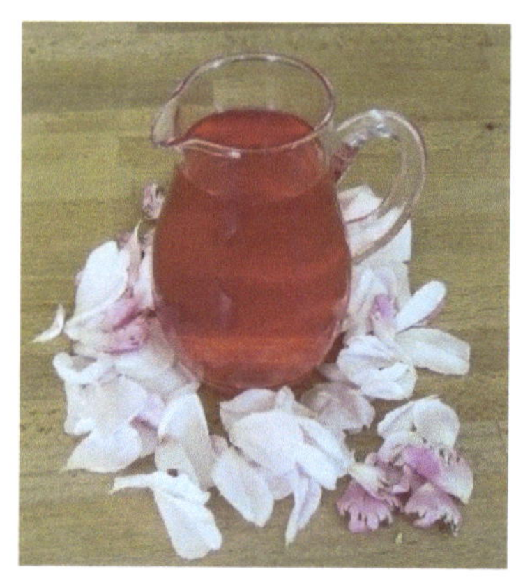

5-6 strongly scented roses (I used a mixture of Apothecary's Rose, William Shakespeare and Gertrude Jekyll)
20 lemon balm stems
4 flowering stems of self-heal
4 lemons
2 lbs of sugar
2 UK pints (20fl oz) of water
Remove the leaves from the lemon balm stems and the leaves and flower stalks from the self-heal and place in a large bowl. Chop into small pieces with scissors. Add all the rose petals and mix. Remove the ends of the lemon and cut into slices. Add these slices to the herbs. Measure the sugar and cold water and place in a saucepan on the heat. Bring to the boil stirring all the time with a long wooden spoon. Pour the sugar syrup carefully into the bowl. Cover with a suitably sized dinner plate so all the plant material is submerged under the syrup. Place the bowl in a cool larder or fridge overnight. You will see that the syrup has turned pink by the following morning. Remove the dinner plate and strain the syrup into a jug. Squeeze the plant material well to remove as much syrup as possible. If you want to maximise your syrup, return the squeezed plant matter to the bowl and cover with cold water. Mix well then strain again and drink. (This should provide your first taste of the cordial at a strength ready for imbibing.)

Pour your rose syrup either into sterilized glass bottles or clean plastic bottles and immediately freeze. The bottles should be sealed, labelled and dated and kept in the fridge once open. Dilute to taste with still or sparkling water.

Mint and lemon balm cordial

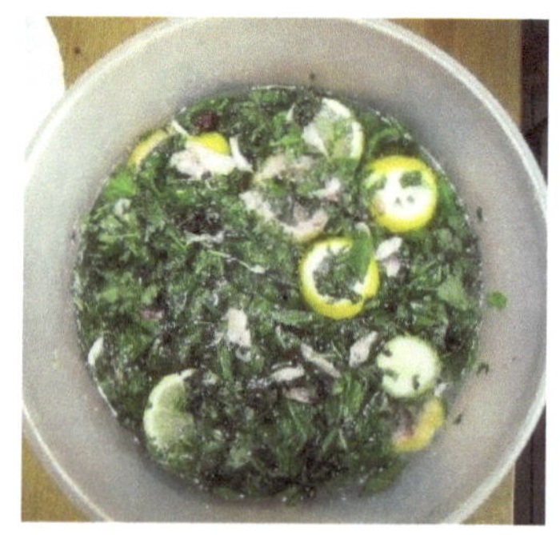

20-30 long stems of mint picked before flowering
10 stems of lemon balm
4 lemons
2 lbs sugar
2 UK pints (20fl oz) of water
Remove leaves from mint and lemon balm, place in a large bowl and chop into small pieces with scissors. Remove the ends of the lemon and cut into slices. Add these slices to the herbs. Measure the sugar and cold water and place in a saucepan on the heat. Bring to the boil stirring all the time with a long wooden spoon. Pour the sugar syrup carefully into the bowl. Cover with a suitably sized dinner plate so

all the plant material is submerged under the syrup. Place the bowl in a cool larder or fridge overnight. Remove the dinner plate and strain the syrup into a jug. Squeeze the plant material well to remove as much syrup as possible. If you want to maximize your syrup, return the squeezed plant matter to the bowl and cover with cold water. Mix well then strain again and drink. (This should provide your first taste of the cordial at a strength ready for imbibing.)

Pour your mint syrup either into sterilized glass bottles or clean plastic bottles and immediately freeze. The glass bottles should be sealed, labelled and dated and kept in the fridge once open. Dilute to taste with still or sparkling water.

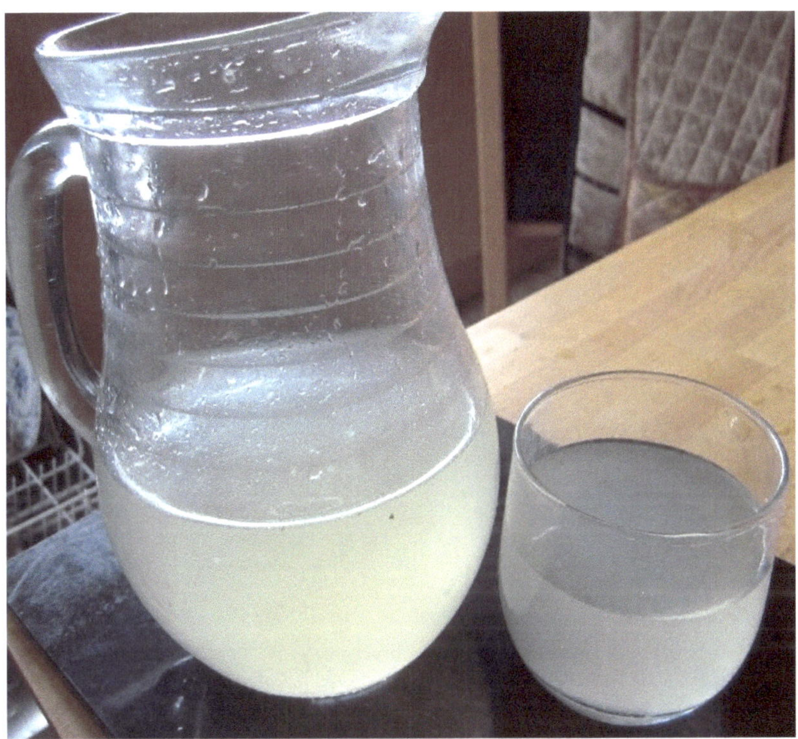

Diluted mint and lemon balm cordial

Notes

Chapter Two

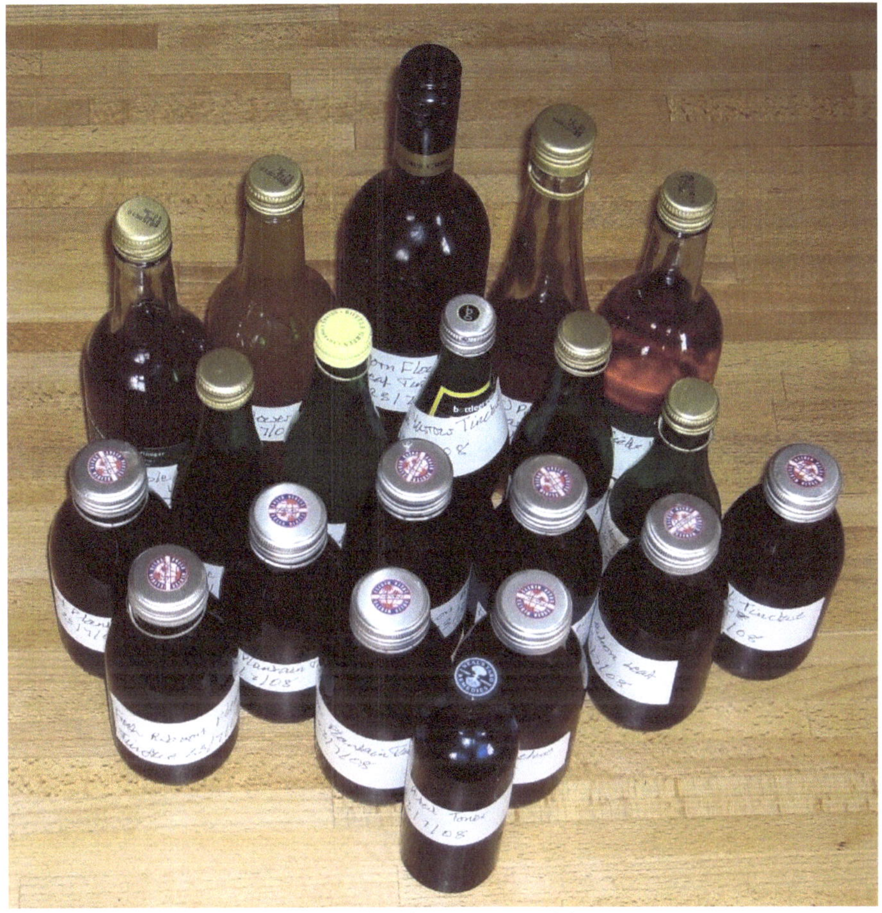

A day's tincture making

Using alcohol

What is a tincture?

Tincture is the name given to the liquid produced when a herb is extracted in alcohol. Each plant is made up of many different chemical constituents and different ones are soluble in different menstrums (liquid mediums). This means some parts dissolve better in water, some in alcohol, minerals in vinegar etc.

Since prehistoric times, herbs have been associated with alcohol. Nettles, alecost, mugwort and meadowsweet have a long history within brewing because they both flavoured the beer and ensured it didn't go bad too quickly. Hops replaced other herbs in brewing during medieval times because they had a greater antiseptic effect on the beer. Stephen Buhner also believes it was the first herbal contraceptive encouraged by the church because hops depress male hormones!

Ancient herbalists, such as Galen and Culpepper talk at length about infusing herbs in wine – mainly because wine was cheap and easily obtainable and patients would be happy to drink their medicine if it came in a form they enjoyed. Some herbs were used to ferment and make into wine, which then had a medicinal effect. Coltsfoot flowers were used for asthma and other bronchial troubles, elderflowers make a cooling champagne for summer while elderberries made a deep rich wine to ward off winter infections.

Tinctures as we know them today are normally made with spirits, rather than wine. The spirit most used in the UK is vodka. This is because the quality of the vodka does not affect its ability to extract the herb, so you can always buy the cheapest brand rather than the most expensive as you would with brandy.

Why use tinctures?

The popularity of tinctures stems primarily from their ease of use. Once made, a tincture can be accessed immediately and used. If you only have a small amount of a certain herb, you can make a tincture from it and increase the doses available compared with making a tea from the same amount of herb. If your herbal harvest is soaking wet when you gather it and there are real fears that it would go mouldy if you put it to dry, you can still make a tincture or vinegar with it, thereby not losing your harvest!

Tinctures are easy to blend into formulas. When you are first learning about herbs, it is probably best to start by using one herb at a time (simpling), but you may wish to combine different herbs to offer particular help. Michael Moore and David Hoffman provide safe, easy to follow formulae for different conditions and Joyce Wardwell has a section in her book, "The Herbal Home Remedy Book", giving general principles of how to combine herbs together.

Tinctures are easy to take with you if you are travelling. They can be kept for a short time in plastic bottles, cutting down on weight. If you are flying, tinctures should be packed in hold baggage and be labelled with printed rather than hand written labels.

There is a danger than tinctures will be confiscated if taken in hand luggage and dried plant material can also be taken from you.

Tinctures can be added to other drinks to enhance medicinal effects or provide a quick beverage if you don't have time to make a herbal tea.

How do you make a tincture?

A spirit will extract both alcoholic and water-soluble constituents of a herb. You can only buy 100% alcohol in the UK if you have a license from the Government and you have to account for every drop you use. Non-license holders should consider what they wish to extract and how much money they wish to pay to do so. Henriette Kress recommends drying a herb before tincturing and using the strongest alcohol you can afford – which would probably be a high strength rum.

If you are using pure alcohol, you must add water to the mixture before you add the herb. The proportions are best found in Michael Moore's table which can be found online at http://www.swsbm.com/ManualsMM/HerbTinct3.txt This is a comprehensive list of herbs which Moore considers extract well in alcohol giving the percentage of alcohol to use and ratio of herb:alcohol as well as the dosage and contraindications.

If you are new to preparing tinctures, percentages and proportions can seem very daunting. If you are making herbal medicines for yourself and your family or friends, there is a simple way which gives fairly consistent results, bearing in mind that the quality/components of a herb will vary year on year depending on growing conditions, amount of sunlight, rain, time of harvest, age and maturity of plant etc.

If you want to make a concentrated tincture, you can dry your herb before tincturing. If you are happy to use fresh plant material, you can either use it straight from picking or leave it to wilt overnight or for 2-4 days, making sure it is not exposed to strong sunlight. Wilting time can be useful to encourage insects to leave your herbs.

To prepare a tincture, fill a screw-top glass jar of any size with your fresh or dried herb. Don't pack the dried herb in too tightly or it will absorb all the liquid and you won't make much tincture. Pour vodka over the herb and "podge" it with a chopstick to get all the air bubbles out, top up the vodka again and screw the lid on firmly.

Leave the jar to stand in a cool, dark place for at least three weeks. If you are using fresh herb, the constituents will pass through to the alcohol by osmosis. If you are using dried material, you need vibration.

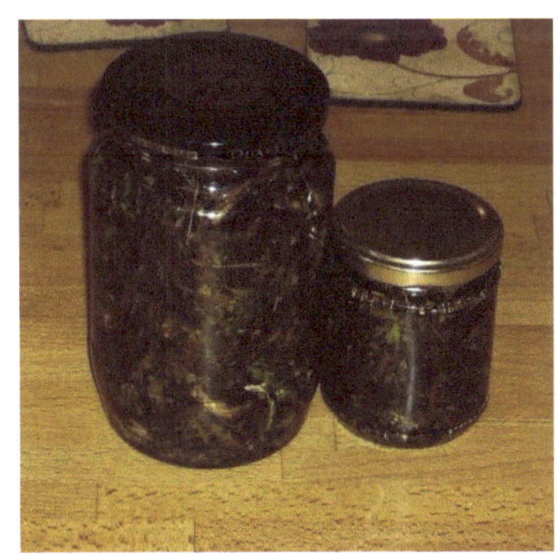

Dandelion root tincture

Shake the bottle every day. When you decide that it has had long enough, decant the

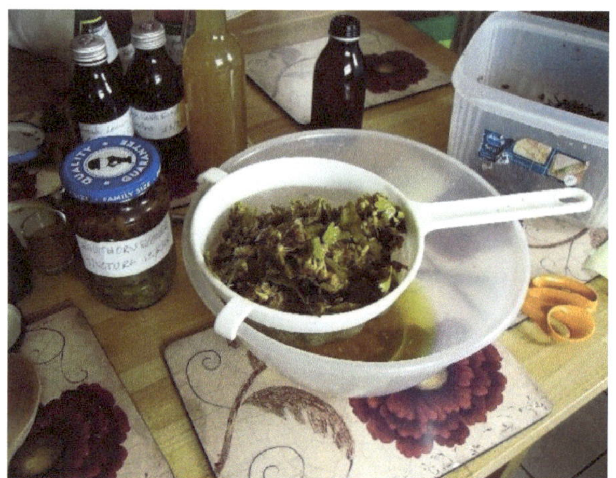

tincture through a plastic sieve into a jug and then pour the liquid into a glass bottle. If the menstrum (i.e. the liquid) is very cloudy, you might want to filter again through a piece of muslin or coffee filter paper. Make sure the bottle top fits securely.

Date and label the bottle so that you know what it is and who made it and when it was made. Tinctures should keep for at least 2 years in a cool dark place, as long as you don't leave the top off and let all the alcohol evaporate.

Decanting hawthorn flower tincture

If you want to reduce the alcohol content of a therapeutic dose of tincture, add boiling water and leave it to cool for at least ten minutes, allowing the alcohol to evaporate.

It is better to make tinctures from single herbs and then mix them with other tinctures rather than try to make a formula with different herbs in the same menstrum.

NB If someone has a compromised or immature liver or an alcohol problem, do not use tinctures. Herbs can be delivered in many other ways such as teas, syrups, vinegars, herbal honey lozenges etc.

Which alcohol should I use?

Some herbs taste better in different kinds of alcohol. Hawthorn berry brandy has a very distinct taste, as has sage brandy. Rum can be useful when extracting very bitter herbs such as motherwort. I use vodka for most of my tinctures and Wray and Nephew's Overproof Rum which is 63% proof for calendula and Solomon's seal root.

Making tinctures with glycerin

Tinctures for children and people who do not wish to use alcohol for medicinal or philosophical reasons can be made by extracting herbs with vegetable glycerin. The resulting tincture is called a glycerite. Glycerin does not extract the same range of constituents from a herb and the body has a 20% less efficiency of absorption in the liver.

Debra St. Claire offers the following comparisons:-

- glycerin will extract the following - sugars, enzymes (dilute), glucosides, bitter compounds, saponins (dilute), and tannins
- absolute alcohol will extract the following - alkaloids (some), glycosides, volatile oils, waxes, resins, fats, some tannins, balsam, sugars, and vitamins.

- glycerin doesn't have the same antiseptic effects as alcohol, so will have a shorter shelf life if fresh plant material is used.

For a simple recipe for making glycerites - mix 75% glycerin with 25% distilled water. Fill a jar with fresh herb, packed to medium density, or fill 1/5 full with dried herb. Pour glycerin menstrum over the herb in the jar. Fill to the top of the jar, covering the plant matter. Label and date. Macerate 2-6 weeks, shaking often (at least once a day). Strain and bottle, label and date. Store in a dark place. The shelf life is said to be 1-3 years, depending upon the water content of the fresh plant used.

A helpful discussion about the benefits of glycerin vs alcohol can be found in this online article http://www.indieherbalist.com/journal/which-is-better-glycerin-vs-alcohol-for-the-best-extracts

Alcohol as preservative

Sometimes it is necessary to add alcohol to a tea to preserve the liquid for longer periods. This is particularly true if you want to make a floral water for cooling hot, inflamed skin or use as a skin cleanser.

Elderflower water

Place elderflowers in a stainless steel or enamel saucepan and cover with fresh spring or distilled water. Cover and slowly heat to just below a simmer. Turn the heat as low as it will go and continue heating for about ten minutes tightly covered. Turn off the heat and allow all to sit, covered, overnight. The next morning, strain the infusion off. You will need to strain at least twice through muslin or kitchen towel to remove all the floating debris. Add a quarter of the volume in alcohol as a preservative. Bottle and keep in a cool dark place.

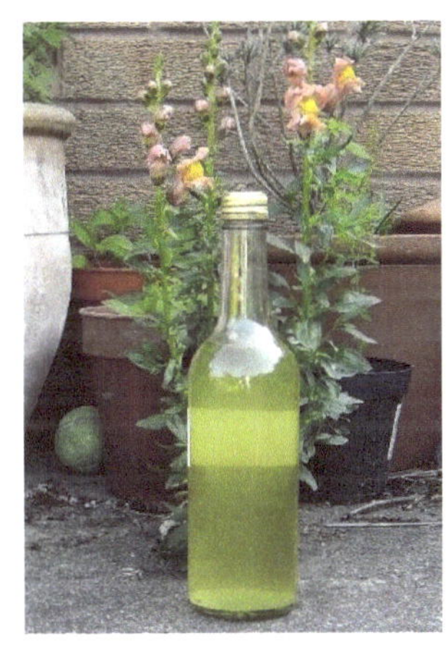

The same recipe can be used to make chamomile water for hot eczema or rose water as a facial cleanser.

Grapefruit bitter aperitif

Slice up some grapefruit peel and remove most of the white pith. Put the slices of peel in a pot with enough water to cover them by about an inch. Add a pinch of salt. Bring the mixture to a boil and simmer it for 15 minutes or so. Drain the peels and set aside the cooking water to make liqueur. Return the peels to the pot, add fresh water, bring it to a boil, and simmer it for another 15 minutes. Drain again (don't forget to save the cooking water).

Bring all the reserved cooking water to a boil and reduce it by about a third. Now add 2/3 cup sugar per cup of water. Stir to dissolve. Let it cool and then add 1 cup of vodka per cup of liquid.

You need to allow plenty of time both for the saved cooking water to reduce and for the sugar water mixture to cool. Pour finished bitter into a glass jar with a screw top lid, label and date. When serving, measure a shot glass full or less and add to fresh grapefruit juice.

Herbal Liqueurs

Herbal liqueurs are basically tinctures where you macerate (soak) a selection of herbs and spices in vodka or brandy for 6-8 weeks in a warm, dark place before straining and adding ½ to 1 cup of sugar, then leaving to mature in a cool, dark place for several years. When making sloe or damson gin, the sugar is added with the pricked fruit in a wine bottle, filling the bottle half full and leaving to mature for 3-4 months in a warm place before decanting. The resultant gin can be drunk immediately either neat or with lemonade.

Lemon Balm Liqueur

1 75cl bottle of vodka
1/2 cup of lemon balm leaves
1 tsp of cloves
1 tsp coriander seeds
1/2 tsp carraway seeds
2 tsps grated lemon rind
3 tsps marjoram leaves

Wash and chop the herb leaves, adding the spirit with the pounded seeds and cloves and grated lemon rind. The cloves should be measured whole, but ground before adding. Leave to steep in a tightly closed jar in a warm dark place, swirling daily for 6-7 weeks. Filter and sweeten to taste with approximately 1/2-1 cup of sugar before labelling in the original bottle and maturing for at least a year. You can use orange peel instead of lemons. You may also wish to reduce the amount of cloves as more than six can result in a medicinal rather than pleasant taste (think mouthwash!).

Rosemary liqueur

1 70cl bottle of brandy
1 tblsp flowering rosemary
3 tsp lavender flowers
8 borage flowers
1 tsp of chopped thyme leaves and flowers
1/2 tsp cloves
1/2 tsp cardoman seeds

The leaves must be stripped from the rosemary stems before washing, drying and pounding them to bring out the flavour. Strip the lavender flowers from their stems before adding and remove the green parts from the borage flowers. Once they have been measured, grind the cloves and the cardamom seeds together and add to all the herbs already in the jar of brandy. Set the labelled and tightly sealed jar in a warm cupboard for six weeks. Try to remember to give the jar a swirl every so often. At the end of this time, filter out the herbs, adding 1/2-1 cup of sugar to sweeten before bottling. Label again and store for at least three to four years.

Hawthorn Liqueur
First, infuse a jar of haws in brandy for three weeks in a cool, dark place. Strain off the liquid and remove the haws. Replace the infused brandy in the jar and add 1 grated nutmeg, one cinnamon stick (crumbled), the chopped peel of one orange, 4 cloves and ½-1 cup full of sugar or honey. Seal the jar with a screw top lid, place in a warm, dark place for 8 weeks shaking regularly, then strain and pour into a sterile bottle. Seal the bottle with a screw top lid or cork and leave in a cold dark place to mature for as long as possible (at least two years).

This recipe was invented after I discovered a glutinous mass in my infused haw tincture. The haws had been collected in December after a frost and the large pectin content caused the precipitation. Rather than throw away the infused brandy, I added sugar and spices and left it to mature. The precipitate disappeared and the resulting liqueur was delicious. I have repeated the recipe several times with haws collected before the frost. The precipitate has not reappeared but the liqueur is just as tasty!

Notes

Chapter Three

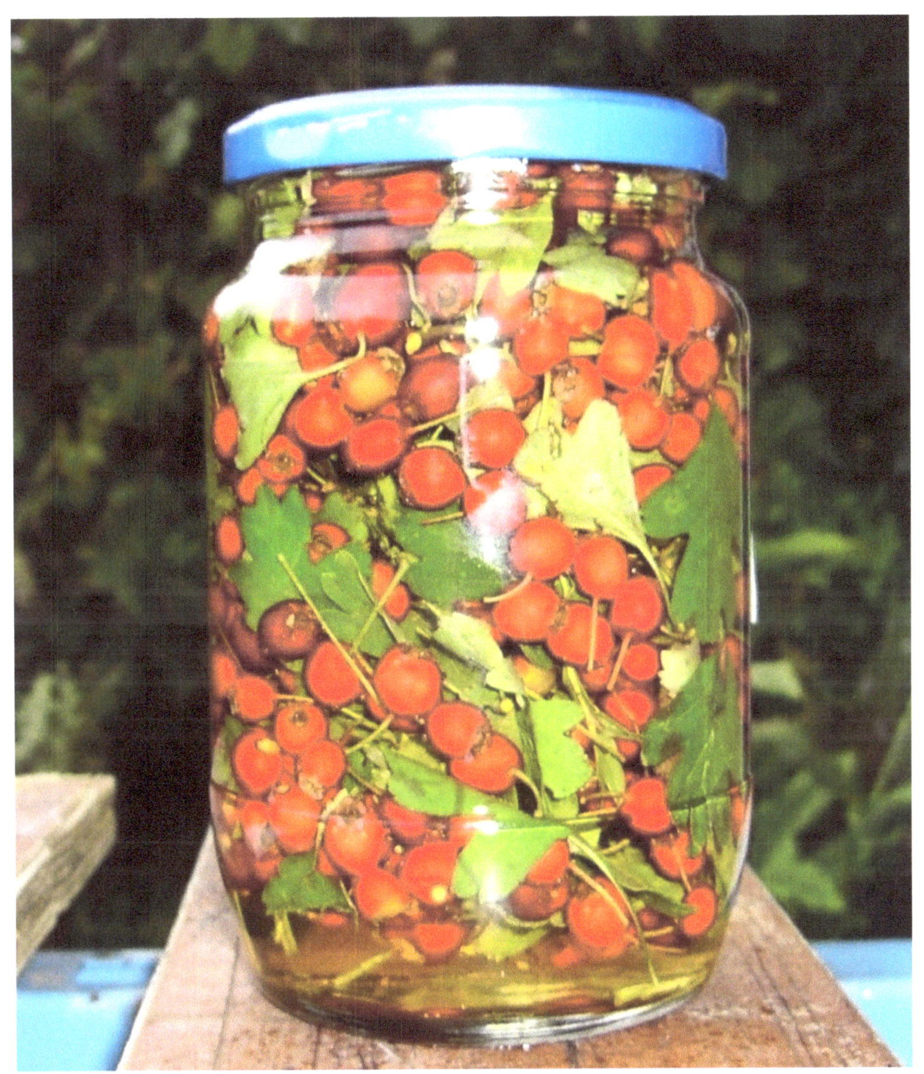

Using vinegar

The word vinegar comes from the French *vin aigre* which means sour wine. Vinegar is formed when alcohol produced by the fermentation of a primary sugar source using yeast goes through a secondary fermentation process. The original sugar source can be anything from molasses, dates, sorghum, fruits, berries, melons, coconut, honey, beer, maple syrup, potatoes, beets, malt, grains to whey. Most commercial vinegars are made either from red or white wine or apples/cider.

A good quality vinegar is a living, breathing entity. Most medicinal vinegars are made from cider vinegar, also known as apple cider vinegar or ACV. You can make your own cider vinegar from any kind of apple or even from cores and peel. Recipes are easy to find and the process can take anything from two weeks to three months depending how strong you wish your vinegar to be.

Commercial vinegars must be at least 4% proof but homemade cider vinegar may be as little as 2%. If you make your own and it is a weaker brew, any herbal vinegars may not last as long. Herbal vinegars made from commercial vinegars can last ten years or more.

It may be helpful to think about the use of your infused herbal vinegar before you make it. If they are destined for a salad dressing you may want to experiment with a variety of base vinegars and concentration of herb to discover your preferred flavour.

Vinegar in cooking

Vinegars can also be very helpful in releasing minerals from bones when making stock. Cover any kind of bones with cold water, add peppercorns, a bay leaf, sprigs of thyme and sage and two tablespoons of cider vinegar. Chopped onions, garlic and celery can also add nutrients. Bring to the boil, simmer for 3-5 hours or more. Strain and either use as a base for soups, sauces or stews or freeze until needed.

Household cleaners

If you are infusing a vinegar to mix with bicarbonate of soda for a cleaning agent, it is best to use white wine or distilled wine vinegar since this will leave no mark on the cleaned surface. Favourite scents are often citrus from grapefruit or orange peels or lavender.

The basic method of making cleaning vinegars is to fill a glass jar with chopped peel or lavender heads, fill with white vinegar, seal and leave to infuse for three weeks in a warm place then strain and use. Such vinegars can also be used instead of fabric conditioners in the washing machine.

Herbal vinegars can also be used as cleansing agents if the infused herb has anti-viral or anti-bacterial properties. Rosemary vinegar on its own can be used to clean your toilet or wash down kitchen surfaces if you want a bacterial wipe. Don't use vinegar if you have previously used bleach or the surface of the bowl will be damaged.

Hair rinse

Use rosemary vinegar as a final rinse in your hair instead of a conditioner. Other herbs will have an affinity for different types of hair such as chamomile for greasy hair.

Making herbal vinegars

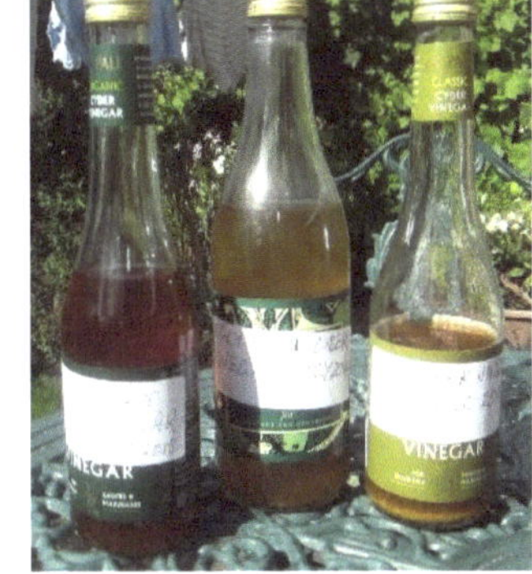

To make a vinegar from fresh herbs, gather on a dry day once the dew has gone from them and shake them to make sure that you are not going to include ants, flies, spiders or other insects in the mixture. Fill a glass jar with the aerial parts and pour cider vinegar over them. You can include stems if they are not too woody, or you might want to use only the leaves and flowers.

Using dry herbs for your vinegars will produce a concentrated macerate. Sometimes there will be seasons when the sun doesn't shine for very long and the only time you have to gather herbs is when they are wet. I have used vinegar as the preferred medium to infuse these wet herbs and have been delighted with the result.

Stir the mixture with a chopstick to bring all the air bubbles to the top (you'll be amazed how air bubbles stick to the leaves) and then seal the lid of the jar tightly. This is to ensure that when you pick the jar up regularly to shake it, the lid doesn't fly off and you end up with herbs and vinegar all over the kitchen! If you are using a metal lid, cover the top of the jar with cling film before sealing to prevent the vinegar from eating the metal.

If you are in a hot climate, you can use the sun to heat your vinegar. Place the vinegar jar in a sunny window or in a greenhouse where the sun can warm it over a period of time. You can strain the vinegar after 3-6 weeks and use it, or leave it as long as you want. You can also use this method to make a vinegar with raspberries, blackberries or hawthorn berries.

You don't need to worry about botulism poisoning when you make herbal vinegars because the toxin cannot live in the acid environment.

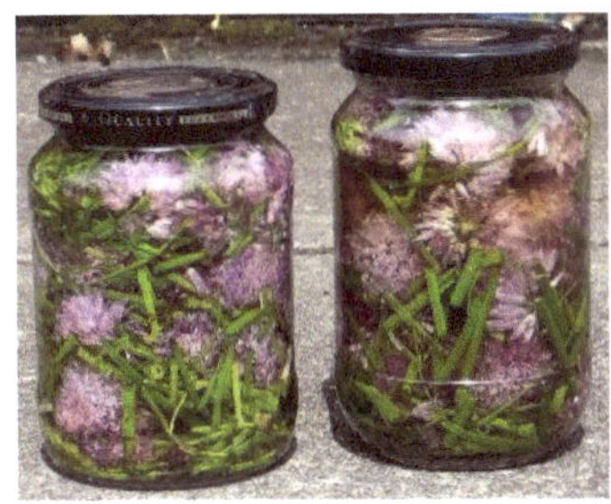

Chive vinegar

If you live where the weather is not reliable, it is probably best to infuse your vinegar in a cupboard which is regularly heated either by water pipes, a hot water tank or radiator. The heat does not have to be strong or continuous but the vinegar does need to be warmed on a regular basis. I have a cupboard where the hot water pipes from my central heating system warm the air even during the summer time when all the heating is off. This is where all my vinegars are macerated.

Medicinal vinegars

Vinegars have been used as medicines since Babylonian times. The ancient healer, Avicenna, used predominantly infused vinegars and honeys to treat his patients. They can be employed in the same way as alcoholic tinctures which makes them invaluable if you do not wish to use alcohol for faith or other reasons.

Table to show Medicinal Properties and Uses of Herbal Vinegars

HERB	PROPERTY	USE
Angelica leaf	Warming, expectorant, tonic	Respiratory infections
Borage	Grounding, adrenal support	Adrenal exhaustion, post viral syndrome
Bramble root	Astringent, carminative	Loose stools, stomach upsets
Chamomile	Anti-fungal, carminative	Fungal infections in hot, airless spaces e.g. groin, behind ears etc.
Dogrose petals	Cooling	To lift the mood, cooling for burns, grief
Elderflower	Anti-viral, cooling,	For fevers, grief, hot flushes, hot joints
Garden rose petals	Cooling, astringent	Burns, household cleanser
Goldenrod	Anti-viral and bacterial, bitter	Useful for children's respiratory infections
Haws	Cardiac tonic, anti-inflammatory, bio-flavanoids	Heart problems, courage, grief, broken heart, savoury sauce for meat
Horseradish root	Anti-congestant, anti-inflammatory	Sinus infections, poultice to warm arthritic joints (may cause blistering on sensitive skin)
Lavender	Nervine tonic, anti-bacterial	Calming, as a cleaning agent to provide peaceful scent
Lovage	Bitter-sweet sedative, aromatic, expectorant, digestive aid, anti-spasmodic, expectorant	Salad dressing, in soups to extract minerals from bones and add flavouring

Motherwort	Supports reproductive system in women, nervine tonic, cooling	Period pains, menopausal problems, stress, grief
Mugwort	Digestive tonic	Use for mineral content in salad dressing, soups etc.
Nettle leaf	High mineral content released into vinegar	Use for osteoporosis prevention
Red Clover	Cooling, alterative, diuretic, expectorant	Use for mineral content, especially with skin conditions, gout, degenerative conditions
Rosemary	Anti-viral, anti-bacterial	Use as household cleanser or hair rinse
Sage	Anti-viral and bacterial	Use for throat and chest infections or soreness, build immunity to hay fever in early part of the year
Winter Savory	Culinary herb	Use for salad dressings etc.
Yarrow	Anti-inflammatory, wound healing, blood dispersal	Use in inflammatory conditions, gout, bruising, viral infections

Vinegars can be combined to provide useful synergies as you would tinctures. Doses can be taken in water or as a hot or cold drink with honey or added to food. If you are using a herbal vinegar as an anti-bacterial or anti-fungal skin wash, remember to dilute the vinegar before using, otherwise it can sting quite badly, especially if the skin is broken.

Oxymels

A mixture of honey and vinegar is often known as an oxymel or honeygar. Some herbalists like to make their oxymels as a single item by adding honey to the infusing vinegar with the herbs. I prefer to keep the two mediums separate until after the infusions have been strained of its plant matter as the honey can promote fermentation, especially where natural yeasts are present. Exploding glass jars are not happy events.

My usual recipe for making a hot oxymel is to mix 2 tsps herbal vinegar with 2 tsps of plain or herbal honey in a mug of boiling water and sip. Sage oxymel is wonderful for soothing sore throats. The powerful anti-viral oxymel made from fire cider vinegar and horseradish honey will kill most viruses stone dead and will certainly clear stuffed noses/unblock sinuses with only three mugs drunk during the day to sleep easily at night.

Mint Sekanjabin is an ancient Arabic cooling drink used to aid digestion. It is made from mint infused vinegar and a delicious mint honey made by macerating mint, grated lemon zest and lemon juice in runny honey for 4-6 weeks.

Mineral rich herbal vinegars

Cider vinegar is the best medium for releasing minerals from herbs such as nettle, oatstraw, motherwort, mugwort, violet leaves or red clover. Motherwort is such a bitter herb that it is difficult to tolerate in a simple tea or tincture but it is enjoyable as an infused vinegar.

To add even more mineral to such a vinegar, wash egg shells in salted water, remove the white membrane from the inside of the shell and dry. Crush the dried shell and add to the macerating herbal vinegar. The vinegar will break down the shells so they are absorbed into the maceration leaving no trace behind. This mineral-rich vinegar can be used for prevention of osteoporosis especially during or post-menopause.

Recipes

Like chai, everyone has their own favourite recipe of fire cider vinegar. In my household, it is the first thing we turn to when a virus hits. As long as you add equal quantities of fresh garlic, horseradish and ginger, the amount of other spices can be left up to the individual. The original recipe did not include rosehips. I've always included them to increase the amount of available vitamin C to help fight infections. If you are in a place where rosehips are not available or are prohibitively expensive to buy, substitute another fruit rich in vitamin C if this is something you feel will be useful.

Fire Cider Vinegar
Equal portions of horseradish and ginger root – grate or whizz in a coffee grinder. (It is your choice whether you peel the roots or not depending on their provenance.)
1 head of garlic, peeled and coarsely chopped
1 good handful of rosehips (fresh or dried)
6 cloves
2 tsps paprika
2 tsps tumeric
2 tsps cayenne pepper
(If you have access to fresh or dried chilies, you can add these as well, leaving the seeds in to give extra "fire"!)

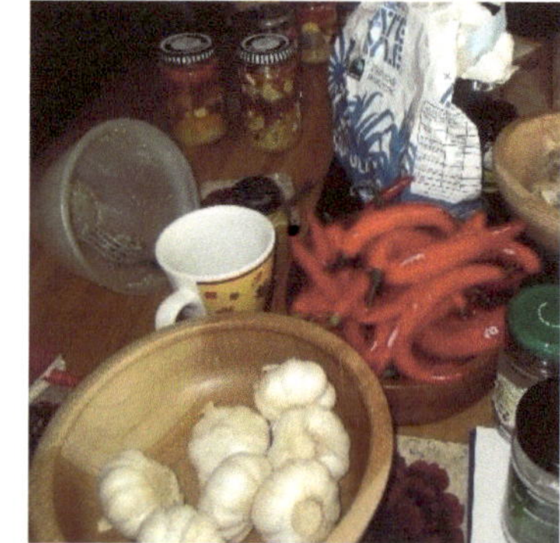

Mix all dry ingredients together in a large glass jar so it is filled about half full, then add cider vinegar, stirring well to remove air bubbles until the jar is full. Place cling film over the top of the jar before sealing with screw top lid. Label and date. Place jar in warm, dark place for 3 weeks. Strain and use. You can reuse the strained material by refreshing with fresh dried spices and infusing in another batch of cider vinegar for three weeks. This second flush will give you a slightly weaker fire cider but it will still be helpful in combatting seasonal ailments.

When the Black Death came to Europe during the Middle Ages and Tudor times, Italian doctors developed an anti-septic vinegar to guard against infection. Mythology tells us it was a group of thieves, stealing from plague-ridden empty houses who used the vinegar to protect themselves. The American herbalist, Karen Vaughan, developed a vinegar based on the "Four Thieves" recipe to protect against respiratory infections.

Thieves Vinegar
1/4 cup dried lavender blossoms
1/4 cup sage
1/4 cup lemon balm
1/4 cup rosemary
1/4 cup peppermint
2 tbsp crushed chilies
2 tbsp cloves
8 minced cloves of fresh garlic
1 fluid oz. wormwood tincture
2 cups apple cider vinegar.
Mix the dried herbs well and place in a jar, along with the garlic. Cover with the tincture and vinegar. Let this sit in a dark place for four weeks, shaking each day. Strain and decant. You can use the infused herbs after straining in soup stock if you wish. Karen said she found that most of the Italian food spices worked well in the vinegar, so don't be afraid to add or substitute with thyme, oregano, zatar, bergamot, or similar anti-infective herbs. (Increase the vinegar proportionally if you add.)

If you suffer with an under-active thyroid, it is a good idea to keep away from horseradish and other brassicas. Some people find horseradish irritates their stomach, so Kiva Rose Hardin developed a different style of infused cider vinegar to aid digestion. It can be taken in many different forms, in soups, salad dressings, spooned on steamed veggies, even marinating meat. The warming, tonic herbs help build and maintain the immune system, increase circulation and generally enhance a sense of well-being. The basil and hawthorn add a relaxing aspect, and the whole infusion is a potent digestive helper.

Gila Harvest Vinegar
1/2 to 3/4 cup fresh turmeric (roughly chopped)
1/2 to 3/4 cup fresh ginger (grated or finely chopped)
1 head fresh garlic (minced)
2-3 tbsp fresh rosemary (roughly chopped)
1 small handful sundried tomatoes (roughly chopped)
2 tbsp coriander seeds (crushed in a mortar and pestle or powdered)
1 small handful dried hawthorn berries (whole)
2 tbsp fresh grated orange peel

3/4 cup fresh basil
1 whole red chili
approximately 3 cups apple cider vinegar
raw honey to taste
1 quart/ 2 pt/1 litre preserving/ Kilner jar
Kiva makes her vinegar in layers, starting with the turmeric and working up to the chili, but you could just as well mix it together beforehand. You can adjust amounts to suit your taste and to properly fill your jar. After you add all the solid ingredients, pour the ACV over the top until the jar is full. Let it macerate for about six weeks.

Strain the cider vinegar, preserving both liquid and herbs. Add honey to taste. You can then refill the jar of preserved herbs with ACV again for a slightly weaker cider vinegar (you can freshen it up with more rosemary and other spices). Or you can put the herbs through the blender with a new batch of ACV and have a more concentrated version.

Sun dried tomatoes and fresh basil are not always available, so this is another recipe I have played around with. It's really nice if you have holy basil growing and can add a large handful of leaves and stems to the mix.

Sarah's digestive vinegar
2 inch root of fresh ginger grated
1 small head of garlic peeled and crushed/chopped
1 large handful of fresh rosemary chopped coarsely
1 large handful fresh or dried rosehips
1 small handful fresh or dried haws
2 tblsp freshly grated orange peel
2 tblsp coriander seeds crushed in a pestle and mortar or ground
1 whole red chili
1 tsp powdered turmeric
Cider vinegar

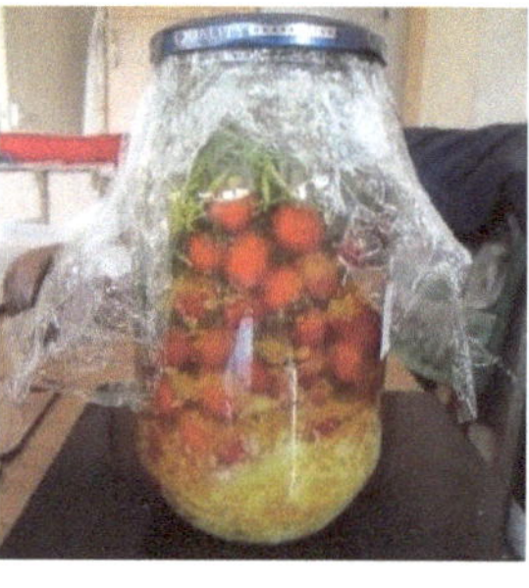

Layer your ingredients in a large glass jar until it is half full then cover with cider vinegar, podging with a chopstick to remove air bubbles then refill with more cider vinegar. Put clingfilm over the mouth of the jar before putting on a metal lid. We strained the infused vinegar after a month and re-used the ingredients after blitzing with more cider vinegar to make another infusion.

Chapter Four

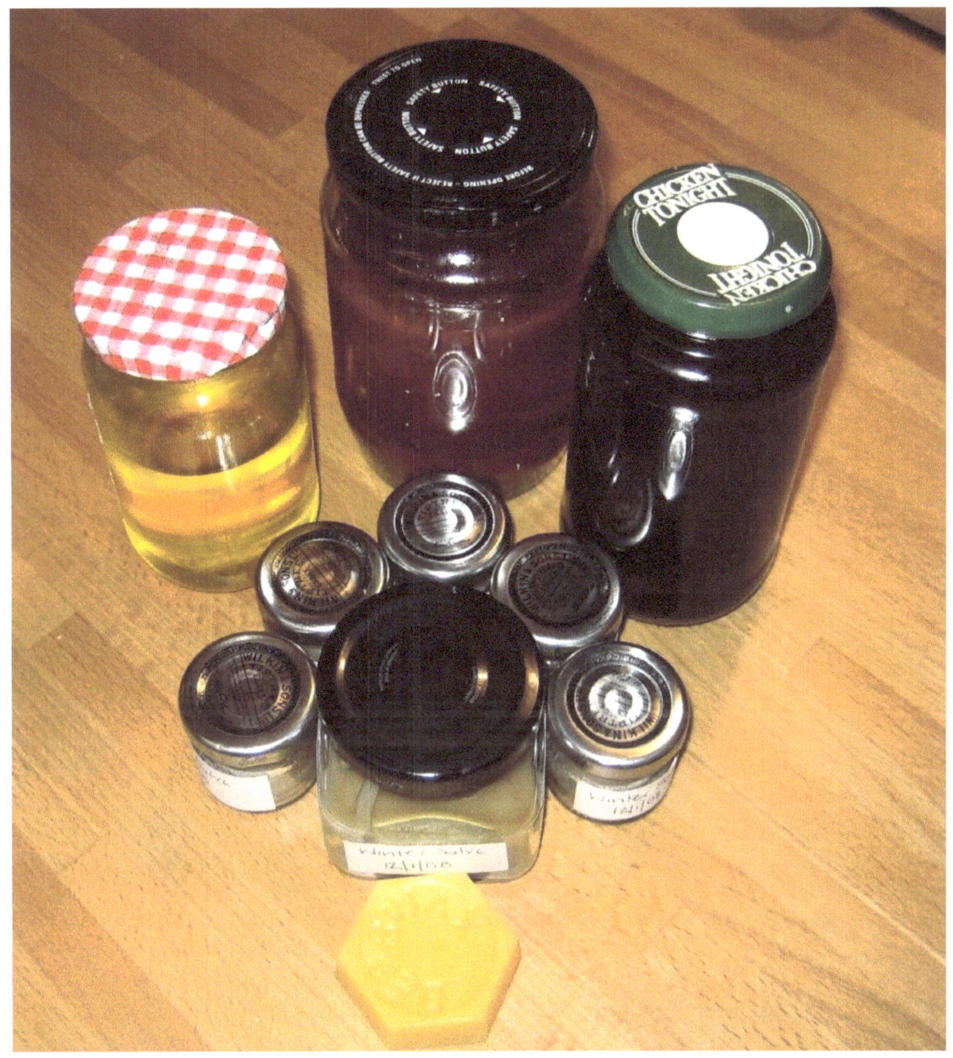

Using Oils

Infused Herbal Oils

Infused oils are very simple to make as long as you have time and patience. There are several different methods of infusion. No one method is right or wrong, each will deliver a desired result but one method may suit a particular herb or climatic condition more than another. You have to experiment and see which method you prefer.

Sun infusion

If you live where large amounts of sunshine are guaranteed, you may be taught to make an infused oil by filling a glass jar with fresh herb (possibly wilted for several hours to reduce the water content), covering the herb with your oil of choice so the entire area of herb is covered and either leaving it in the sunshine or another suitable warm place for six weeks or burying it in hot sand/earth overnight or for several days. The only drawback to this method is that if you leave any part of the herb exposed to the air, or if you seal the jar tightly so water vapour from the fresh plant material cannot evaporate, mould may form or the oil may become rancid so that at the end of the six weeks you have to throw everything away. You need to check the oil regularly to ensure everything is okay.

The only herb I infuse by the sun method is St John's wort. The first blooms appear on or around the summer solstice. I pick the flowers either daily or every few days, place them in a glass jar and cover them with sunflower oil. St John's wort is a very delicate flower and needs a very light oil. The jar is then placed, uncovered, on my kitchen window sill until the 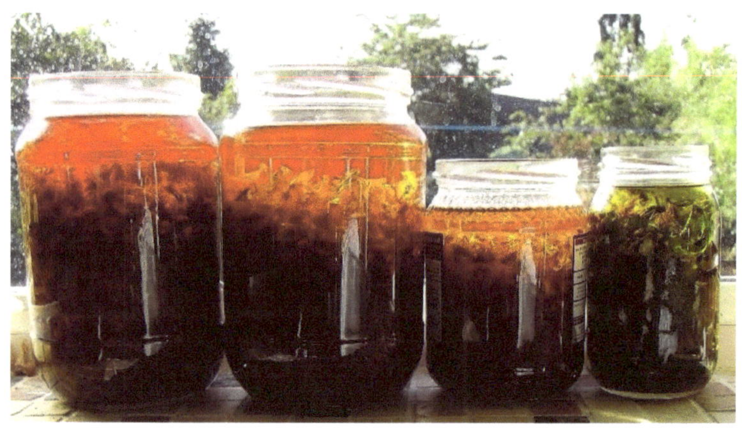 end of September, early October when I strain out the plant material and place the infused oil in a clean jar, seal and date.

The jar is left uncovered to ensure the water vapour from the flowers can evaporate. You can put a lid on as long as it isn't sealed, but I have had problems with doing this. If you are worried that flies or other insects might contaminate your oil, you can cover it with a cotton/linen jug cover or a small piece of butter muslin/cheesecloth.

St John's wort oil can be made cumulatively. If you only have a small amount of flowers, these can be placed in a jar and covered with oil, then a further harvest can be added to the jar on further occasions until the jar is full. The oil will start turning colour after 4-7 days, gradually changing colour from yellow to pale pink to deep crimson as the active constituents of the plants are released into the oil. It will also take on a distinctive aroma, which is unique to St John's wort oil.

Double infused external heating method

While the sun infused method of making herbal oils is popular in the United States, European herbalists usually prefer to heat their herbs using the double infused method on a stove/cooker using the principles of a bain marie/water bath so the oil of choice does not come in to direct contact with the heat source.

The term, "double infused" means that you use the same amount of oil for two separate amounts of herb. This usually means dividing your herb harvest into two piles which you add to the oil at different times, the first amount being added at the beginning and the oil then being strained and the first portion removed at the end of the required time, then the strained oil is poured over the second portion which is subsequently heated.

If you are intending to use the infused oil as a massage oil or salve for children or frail elders, you may wish to undertake a single infusion for some highly aromatic herbs e.g. rosemary.

For the classic double boiler double infusion method, you need
- 4 oz./100g fresh or dried herb
- Enough oil to cover half the amount of herb (around 8 fluid ounces/270ml)
- Water
- Either a double saucepan or a stainless-steel pot with a lid small enough to place inside another saucepan.

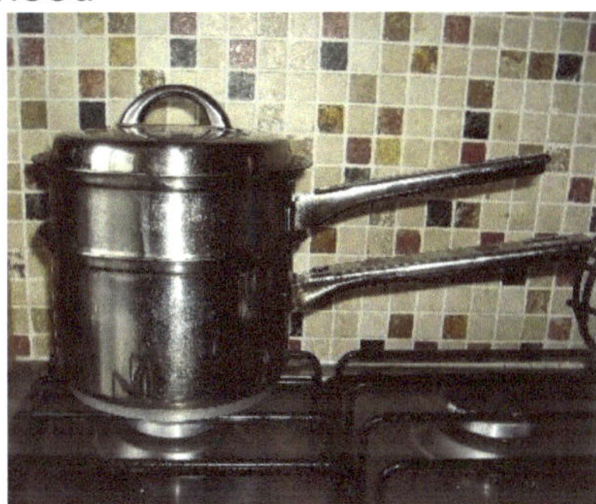

Double boiler saucepan

Place half of the herb inside the inner pan and cover with the oil. Replace the lid firmly and place inside the other saucepan which is about half filled with water. Heat the external saucepan so that the water gently boils. **Do not let the pan boil dry!** Boil for about 2 hours, then remove the inner pan and strain off the oil, compressing the herb if you can to remove as much oil as possible. Place the rest of the herb inside the inner

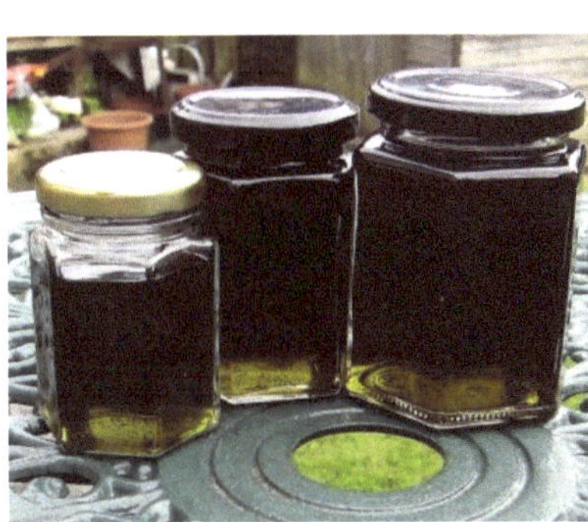

pan and pour over the oil from the first infusion. Replace the lid firmly and heat the oil in the outer pan for a further two hours. Strain the oil into a heated glass bottle or jar and cap with a screw top lid. If using fresh herb, let the infused oil sit for about three days to make sure any water content separates out. Decant oil. If water drops are left in the infused oil it will go off more quickly. Label the oil with the name and date that you made it.

Double infused fresh yarrow oil

The need to weigh and measure your quantities of herb and oil is entirely up to you.

<u>Cookpot/crockpot method</u>

You can heat your oil in a cookpot/crockpot on the lowest setting. You then have the choice of altering the timings and maybe heating overnight for a concentrated single infusion, or for two extended lengths of time for a double infusion.

Remember that oil heats at a temperature higher than water and if you are using fresh plant material, the water vapour will evaporate and collect on the inside of the crockpot lid. Be very careful when removing the lid. Try to lift it up and away quickly so the water droplets do not fall into the hot oil. If this happens, the hot oil can splash and burn you. (I have done this - it's painful!)

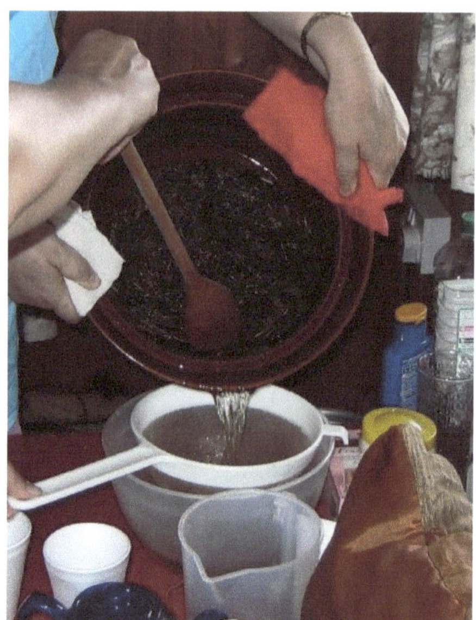

It can be easier to put a closed container inside a cookpot and turn it into a bain marie/water bath. This way it is easier to prevent the infused oil from overheating. You can use a large jam jar as your container if you start the water from cold.

Fresh herbs or dry?

Some people advocate using fresh herbs for infused oils and others prefer to dry them first. If you use fresh herbs, the oil will contain a certain amount of watery matter which can make the oil go bad if not removed before storage.

Removal can be achieved by firstly noticing the globules of water at the very bottom of the infused oil when you are pouring the final straining and leaving it in the pan. The oil can then be left for up to three days to ensure the oil and water layers have separated, then decanting the oil again before final storage.

I have had one occasion when making a double infused fresh rosemary oil in a cookpot, where the resulting infused oil came out as an emulsion and took several months before the oil and water levels separated.

The presence of an aqueous (water) component to an oil does expose it to the danger of botulism being present, since the organism lives in water. The botulin toxin is not destroyed by heat so, if it is present, it cannot be removed. The danger of botulism is rare. I have never heard of a case relating to an infused herbal oil in any country and if your oils are only used externally there should not be a problem. You may wish to make lip balm from oils prepared from dry herbs as the botulin cannot live without water.

If you dry your herb before infusing, there is no water component to worry about but you may feel that the herb is compromised energetically. There are some herbs which are recommended to be dried before infusing into oil because of their resinous quality. Calendula is one of these herbs and is the only herb I deliberately dry before infusing. I do make oils from other dried herbs during the winter if I need to make oils and fresh herbs are not available.

Single or multiple herbs?

It is usually advisable to make an infused oil with a single herb, then mix the infused oils together in desired combinations when putting together a massage oil or salve. If you know which combinations you want to use, you could put them together in the oil, or if you have limited amounts of material, you could do a single infusion of each, but the concentration of each herb will not be as great as preparing a single herb double infused oil.

Which oil?

The type of oil you use to prepare an infused herbal oil depends on your preference and the availability and cost of your preferred medium. Vegetable oils are the most popular medium. Sunflower, safflower, olive, almond, avocado, jojoba and coconut are only a few examples of what is available. You will need to decide what you want to use and what you are prepared to pay for it.

In ancient times, animal fats were the most widely available form of oil and these were used for infused oils as well as lighting. "Leaf tallow" from around the kidneys of an animal is the purest form of fat. It is easily absorbed through the skin and is gaining popularity amongst herbalists who wish to use organic, local, sustainable oils with respect. Beef, mutton, pork, emu and bear fat are all suitable. If carefully rendered and kept in a cool, dark environment, the infused oil can keep without unwanted scent or deterioration for up to a year or more.

Storage

Infused oils should be kept in a cool dark place. If stored correctly they should keep their efficacy for at least two years or more if they remain unopened. You can usually tell if an oil has gone rancid or has no usefulness by the smell/scent. If an oil loses its scent but does not smell unpleasant, it is probably best to discard and make some more.

Salves

Oils are slippery and may be difficult to rub in. You may find it easier to make the infused oil with an oil which is solid at room temperature such as cocoa butter or coconut oil, especially if you don't want to use beeswax. Shea butter is another vegetable oil which is solid, but melts at body temperature.

You may need to use a combination of solid and liquid oils to ensure you get a suitable consistency. If you are using cocoa butter, the combination is 2/3:1/3 of cocoa butter to sunflower oil.

To make a simple salve, grate up some beeswax and add it to the hot infused oil, stirring continuously until it melts. (About 1oz/25g beeswax to 8 fl. ozs/300ml of oil)

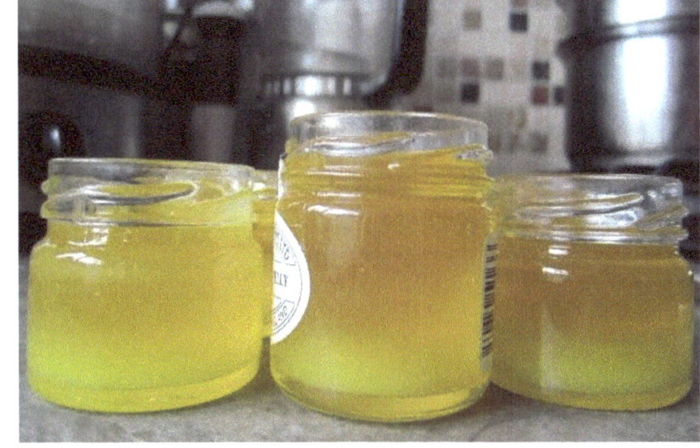

Dandelion salve cooling and solidifying

Test on the back of a wooden spoon to see whether it is of a suitable consistency then pour into small jars and seal. If you are not confident to do the spoon test, an easier way of checking is to drop a very small amount of oil plus melted wax into cold water in a small bowl or mug. The salve will immediately cool and you can rub it between your fingers to check the desired thickness.

The salve will thicken on cooling, usually from the bottom upwards if you pour into cold jars. It will usually be a paler colour than the original oil. St John's wort salve is pink, comfrey salve pale green and dandelion salve pale yellow.

'Rosebud Lips' Balm
225ml (9 fl oz) calendula oil
3 tblsp jojoba oil
45g (1½ oz) dried alkanet root
30g (1oz) beeswax
12 drops rose essential oil (optional)
Gently heat both oils in the top of a double boiler for about 10 minutes. Remove from the heat, add the alkanet root and steep for around 30 minutes, to extract the colour from the root. Strain the root from the oils through a muslin cloth. Return the oils to the double boiler with the beeswax. Once this has melted, remove from the heat and add the rose essential oil drop by drop. Pour into small sterilised pots or jars. Allow to cool thoroughly before putting the lids on.

The whole aim of both infused oils and salves is to deliver a dose of herbal medicine through the body's largest organ, the skin. To improve the transfer through the skin, some herbalists add extra contents such as lanolin or honey. If you decide to experiment with these substances you must ensure the recipient is not allergic to the addition and is not diabetic. Lanolin and honey are both watery substances, so the resulting cream must be thoroughly emulsified before storing and may need to be remixed before applying.

Essential oils

Essential oils can be added to salves to improve their keeping (vitamin E can be used in the same way) or to add scent. Use the least number of drops possible per fluid ounce of salve and never more than four. If your salve is going to a household where young children live or visit, do not include any essential oil.

If you are skilled in aromatherapy, you will know how to use essential oils safely.

Creams

Creams and ointments are made by emulsifying a mixture of infused oil and water. You can also make a cream by adding your own tincture and oil to a commercially prepared cream or ointment.

Christopher Hedley's basic cream recipe
1oz base cream
1 tsp infused oil (e.g. marigold or St John's wort)
2 tsp tincture (e.g. rose petal or comfrey)
4 drops of essential oil (e.g. lavender)
First add the infused oil to the base cream and stir until it is all absorbed. Then add the tincture and stir again, then add the drops of essential oil and stir again. Spoon into small jars with screw top lid and use.

Simple Rose Cream
8 fl ozs Apothecary's rose petal double infused oil
1 fl oz aloe vera gel scraped from the inside of three large leaves
5 fl ozs Apothecary's rose petal tincture
1oz grated beeswax
Measure the oil and heat in the top of a double boiler with the grated beeswax, stirring gently with a wooden spoon until it melts. Pour this liquid into a large plastic bowl suspended inside another bowl of cold water and stir the oil until it is almost cool. Use a stick blender to emulsify the cooling salve whilst slowly pouring the tincture and aloe vera gel into the mixture. Continue blending until the cream is thoroughly emulsified. It should look pale and fluffy and slightly pink in colour. Spoon into sterilized jars with a teaspoon making sure to eliminate any air bubbles. Seal, label and date. Use within three months and keep refrigerated once opened if using several times a day.

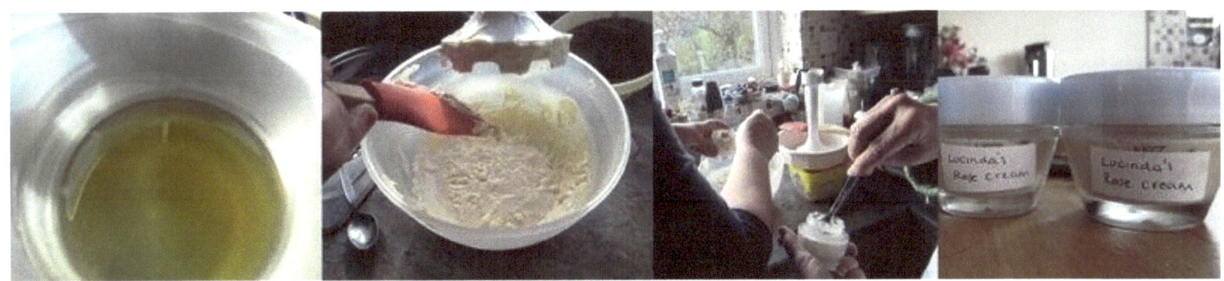

Properties of Herbal Oils

Herb	Medicinal Use	Notes
Agrimony	Use for pain caused by constriction	
Angelica	Use as a skin lotion for itching, wounds and rheumatism, a warming herb	
Calendula	Cracked skin, cuts, chilblains, sunburn, acne, tired feet, inflammations, eczema, has an affinity with skin	
Chickweed	Use to soothe eczema or other itchy conditions	
Comfrey	Use to heal broken bones, sprains and damaged tissues (do not place directly on broken skin)	
Dandelion flower	Use to massage swollen and aching breasts. Helpful for mastectomy scar tissues and light muscle pain massage	
Elderflower	Cooling herb, use on inflamed joints or in a nourishing oil as a face cream	
Elder leaf and bark	Elder leaf and bark can be infused for a bruise oil. Leaf oil makes an effective insect repellant especially when mixed with herb Robert and a few drops of citronella essential oil	
Ginger	Warming oil, use for arthritic aches, joints, improves circulation	

Golden Rod	Anti-inflammatory, anti-microbial, analgesic. Use for deep muscle massage for pain	
Heartsease	Mucilaginous herb, use to moisten and sooth dry inflamed skin, such as eczema	
Herb Robert	Use as general insect repellent, also against headlice.	
Lovage	Use in combination with calendula, St John's wort & marshmallow for tissue lubrication	
Marshmallow	Mucilaginous herb. Use to lubricate and sooth tissues	
Meadowsweet	Anti-inflammatory, analgesic Rub into inflamed joints or other areas to reduce pain	
Mugwort	Rub into inflamed joints or other areas to reduce pain (*NB Do not use on people with allergies*)	
Mullein	Use for ear infections where eardrum is intact or rub below ear. For greatest effect infuse in St John's wort oil.	
Nettle	Use to stimulate hair growth in male and female alopecia. Can also use externally for antihistamine effects.	
Plantain	Drawing herb: use to draw splinters, glass, bee stings and other bites. Use as 'knit-bone' in place of comfrey, to heal old woundsand bruising.	

Rosemary	Use as massage oil for reducing arthritic and sciatic pain	
St John's Wort	Apply to bruises, wounds in danger of infection, burns, ulcers, earache in children (where eardrum intact), anywhere with minor nerve damage e.g. shingles, sciatica,	
Solomon's Seal	Use for joint pain, especially back, shoulders and knees. Combines well with agrimony	
Southernwood	Repels insects	
Tansy	Repels insects	
Vervain	Use in poultice for wounds and burns.	
Violet	Mucilaginous herb, use for dry skin, eczema, to moisturise. Used for ringing in the ears	
Wormwood	Use oil to treat gout and rheumatism. Use with equal parts of groundsel and fresh elderflowers to make oil for bruising and inflammation.	
Yarrow	Use for bruising, old wounds, stagnant blood, anti-inflammatory	

Chapter Five

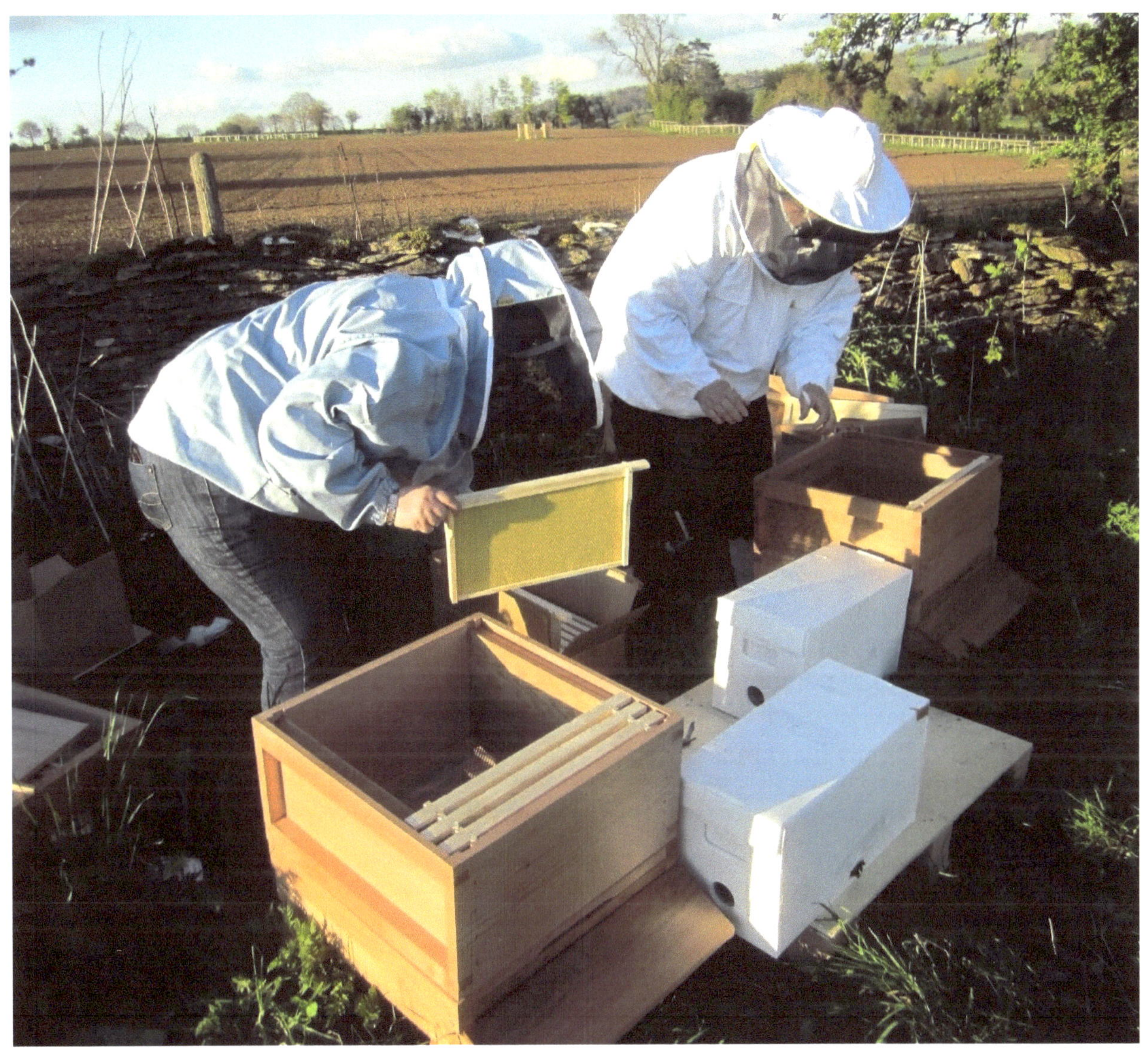

Using Honey

Herbs come in many shapes and forms. Sometimes the flavour is too unpalatable to be easily taken. This is where a source of sweetness can be helpful. Before sugar was freely available, honey and sweetness from naturally occurring fruits were used. In this pamphlet, the properties of honey and ways of using it are discussed.

If you have ethical difficulties in using honey, you may wish to explore the use of other natural sugars or nut butters as alternatives. These cannot be used to extract herbal properties in the same way but they can be used in the production of syrups, electuaries and elixirs.

If you suffer with diabetes or insulin resistant conditions, it is not advisable to use honey, sugar or fruit sugars in any form.

Honey

Honey bees are unique in not hibernating like their wasp and bumblebee cousins. The reason they can survive through the winter is down to the honey they produce from the nectar gathered from flowers. They also huddle together for warmth and keep active.

Honey is a complex mix of:
- 82.4% natural sugars
- 17.1% water
- 0.5% minerals, vitamins, pollen and protein

Of honey's 82.4% natural sugar content, around 70% is made up of fructose and glucose. The balance of these two sugars determines whether a honey is clear or set. The higher the fructose content, the longer the honey will remain liquid. There is no difference in the taste or nutritional value between clear and set honey. Honey can be restored to liquid simply by standing it in warm water for an hour or so or microwaving for thirty seconds.

The flavour, colour and consistency of honey varies, depending on the flowers where the nectar was collected. As a general rule, the darker the colour, the stronger the flavour of the honey.

Honey contains small amounts of a wide range of vitamins and minerals (including iron, potassium, zinc, magnesium, niacin and riboflavin), amino acids and antioxidants. Generally, darker honeys contain higher levels of antioxidants then lighter honeys.

The oldest recorded honey was found in the tomb of an Egyptian couple, Yuya and Tjuyu, by archaeologists, Quibell and Davis, in 1905. It was still recognisable by its scent three thousand years after being placed amongst the burial goods. We know from ancient texts that honey was not only eaten, but used as a medium for herbal medicines wherever a physician could harvest honey from wild or farmed sources.

During the 20th century, use of honey in herbal medicines fell from favour. Many herbalists felt their patients should be exposed to the unadulterated flavours of all herbs in order to counteract the bland and over-sweet diet of most western nations. In more recent years there has been a movement to reduce the reliance on alcoholic herbal extractions and honey is once more being offered as an effective medium for herbal medicines.

Honey on its own has medicinal properties. It soothes sore throats and it is said that taking 1 teaspoon 3 times a day 30 minutes before eating will kill candida. Recent research has confirmed its effectiveness in treating burns, deep wounds and hospital acquired infections.

When I was working in the NHS, I once sat next to a retired practice nurse during a conference dinner, who told me how she used to successfully coat resistant leg ulcers with honey before her managers found out and insisted she used "modern techniques" which never worked as well.

Burns and Honey

The general UK advice about treating burns says

- **Stop the burning process** as soon as possible. This may mean removing the person from the area, dousing flames with water or smothering flames with a blanket. Do not put yourself at risk of getting burnt as well.
- **Remove any clothing or jewellery** near the burnt area of skin. However, don't try to remove anything that is stuck to the burnt skin because this could cause more damage.
- **Cool the burn with cool or lukewarm water** for 10 to 30 minutes, ideally within 20 minutes of the injury occurring.
  - Never use ice or iced water as this can cause further damage
  - Never use creams or greasy substances such as butter as this traps heat
- **Keep yourself or the person warm**. Use a blanket or layers of clothing, but avoid putting them on the injured area. Keeping warm will prevent hypothermia, where a person's body temperature drops below 35ºC (95ºF). This is a risk if you are cooling a large burnt area, particularly in young children and elderly people.
- **Cover the burn with cling film**. Put the cling film in a layer over the burn, rather than wrapping it around a limb. A clean clear plastic bag can be used for burns on your hand.
- **Treat the pain from a burn with** paracetamol **or** ibuprofen. Always check the manufacturer's instructions when using over-the-counter (OTC) medication. Children under 16 years of age should not be given aspirin.

What this advice doesn't tell you is anything to aid the cooling or healing process. Nor does it identify first (reddened skin) or second (blisters) degree burns but only tells you when to head for hospital for
- large or deep burns – any burn bigger than the affected person's hand
- full thickness burns of all sizes – these burns cause white or charred skin
- partial thickness burns on the face, hands, arms, feet, legs or genitals – these are burns that cause blisters
- all chemical and electrical burns

Also get medical help straight away if the person with the burn:
- has other injuries that need treating
- is going into shock – signs include cold clammy skin, sweating, rapid shallow breathing and weakness or dizziness
- is pregnant
- is over 60 years of age
- is under five years of age
- has a medical condition such as heart, lung or liver disease, or diabetes
- has a weakened immune system (the body's defence system), for example because of HIV or AIDS, or because they're having chemotherapy for cancer

If you feel confident to treat the burn at home, make sure you cool the burned skin in water for twenty minutes or more then move on to other treatments if there is continued pain and discomfort. The best agent to continue cooling is aloe vera gel, obtained by removing a fleshy leaf from the plant and slicing it in half, laying the inside straight against the burn. Replace the aloe vera every two hours or so.

It is really important NOT to treat a burn with any oil or salve until ALL the heat has gone. This is because oil traps heat underneath the application.

If you don't have any aloe vera plants or juice then look to other cooling herbs such as elderflower, rose, chamomile, bergamot (preferably wild *monada fistulosa).* These can be applied as a tea, herbal water or diluted infused herbal vinegar.

If the burned skin blisters, try a honey poultice. You can daub honey straight onto the skin and protect it with clingfilm or a cloth bandage covered with something waterproof (to protect clothing) or you can mix the honey with herbal oil derived from those herbs which have an affinity for skin healing and burns such as St John's wort and calendula and then apply to the skin. Leave this honey poultice in place for twelve to twenty-four hours before removing or replacing. You should find the blister has completely disappeared and healing has begun by the second or third day.

If you are concerned the burn may become infected, an infused "burns" honey can be applied. Traditionally the honey is made by gathering three different herbal flowers during the summer and infusing them for six weeks. The honey can then be strained if desired or left in the honey.

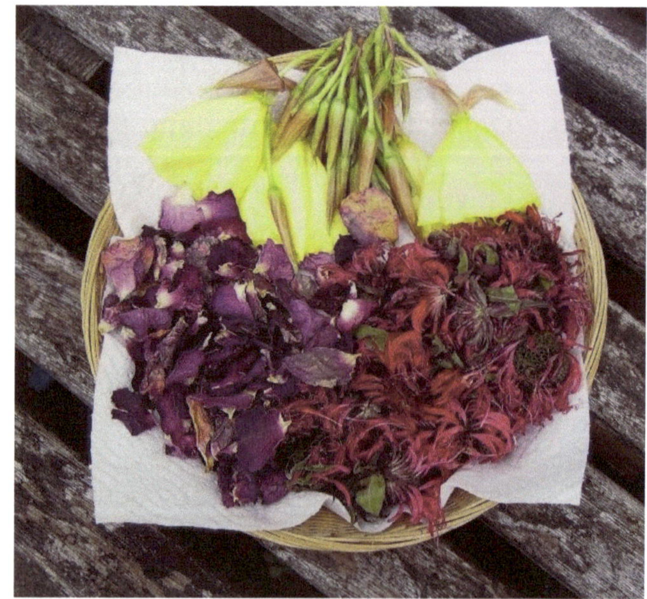

Flowers of apothecary's rose, evening primrose and bergamot

"Burns honey" was first developed by the American herbalist, Kiva Rose Hardin in 2008. She used three local herbs for her honey; bergamot as an anti-viral, antibacterial, apothecary's rose for cooling and evening primrose for cooling and moisturising. We have changed the formula slightly by using St John's wort flowers instead of the bergamot and adding calendula.

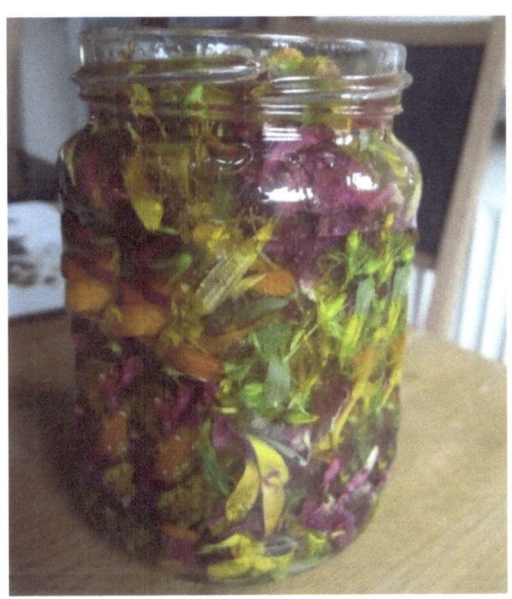

Flowers of St John's Wort, calendula, evening primrose and apothecary's rose in local honey

Remember that burns can take up to two weeks to heal, depending on the severity of the burn and the healing power of the individual. Once healing begins, you can continue treatment by applying salves made from skin-healing herbs twice a day.

Honey as sweetener
Honey can be used as a sweetener in herbal teas. Much smaller amounts are needed than sugar and the flavour of the herb will often be enhanced.

Syrups and cordials

Honey can also be substituted in syrup or cordial recipes for sugar in equal amounts.

Derbyshire Delight

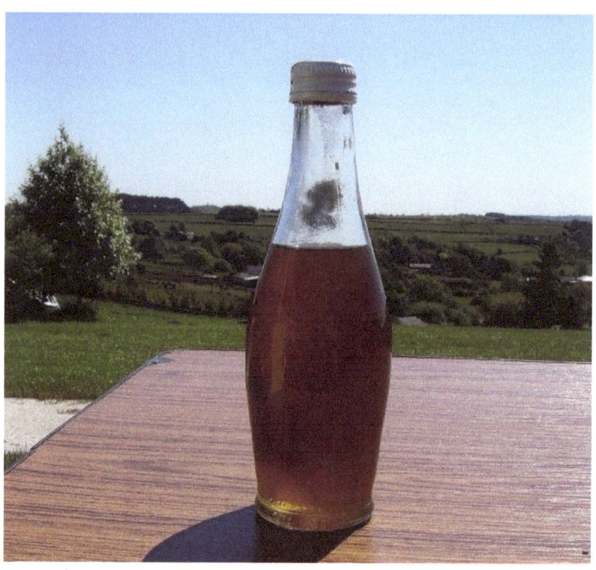

This syrup was first developed whilst on holiday in the Peak District

Pick an amount of fresh dandelions, red clover flowers and stalks and hawthorn flowers. Remove the dandelion petals and centres from any green bits. Place in a saucepan and cover with cold water. Bring to the boil and simmer gently for 20 minutes. Strain and measure liquid. Clean saucepan. Return liquid to the pan and simmer with the lid off until the liquid is reduced by 7/8s. Add honey in the ratio of 1pint/1litre to1lb/1kg honey. Stir gently until honey is dissolved. Pour into heated, sterilized bottles. Seal when cold. Label and date.

Infused honey

When I first started working with herbs, I saw honey only as a sweetener, something to substitute for sugar. It took thirteen years before I became caught up in the enthusiasm of American herbalists and started to experiment with honey as a medium in its own right.

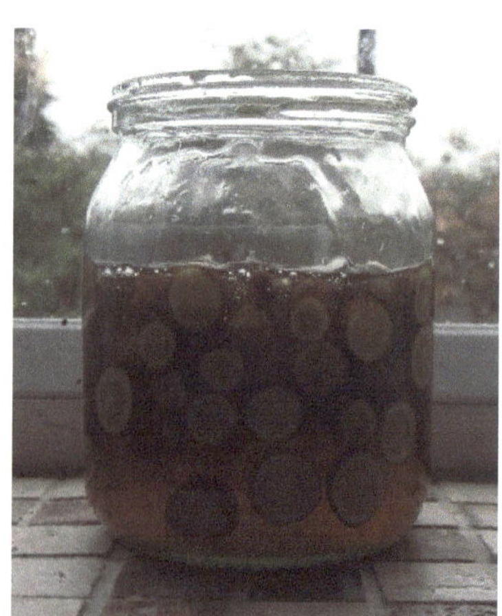

Elecampane root honey

Honey can be used as an extraction medium for herbal medicine or for culinary use. Herbal honeys are easily made by filling a glass jar with fresh leaves, fruits, flowers or washed, sliced or chopped roots and covering with runny honey slowly, removing air bubbles with a chopstick until the jar is full. It is important that all air is removed because it might harbour air-borne bacteria. The honey can then be left to infuse for 4-6 weeks before decanting.

Care must be taken if a herb is covered with natural yeast that a fermentation process does not start. Elderberries are best infused in the fridge unless you want your shelf dyed a fetching shade of purple!

If you are infusing flowers in a honey, don't be surprised if all the plant material gathers at the top of the jar. You can shake it up or even turn the jar on its lid but you may find the honey leaks if you do this. After infusion, you may find the honey is thinner than it was before due to the water content of the flowers.

Kiva Rose Hardin shared a recipe for making an aromatic mint and lemon infused honey. Like other infused honeys, you fill a jar with mint leaves, add 2 teaspoons of grated lemon rind and the juice of one lemon. This recipe is part of an ancient Arabic cooling drink used to aid digestion called Mint Sekanjabin. It is made from mint infused vinegar and the mint honey.

Rosehips can be finely chopped in a food processor before covering with honey, but it is advisable to remove the seeds and seed hairs if you want to be able to eat the honey without straining it. Rosehip seeds are very stony and can break your teeth if chewed inadvertently! Having said that, the flavour is wonderful!

Honeys can be made from all parts of a plant providing they have an aromatic component. Members of the mint family can be the most effective. Here are some examples.

Flowers   marjoram, rose, thyme, evening primrose, self heal, wild bergamot
              (purple), bergamot (red), St John's wort

Leaves   Mint (peppermint/Swiss mint/spearmint/apple mint), sage

Fruit   elderberry, rosehip

Roots/corms   horseradish, angelica, elecampane, garlic, onion

I've noticed that herbs alter the consistency and the sweetness of honey. Using fresh herbs makes the honey thinner because of their water content and a bergamot/ rose/ evening primrose combination is much less sweet.

Everyone thought I was mad mixing grated horseradish with honey until they tried it. The result is a perfect accompaniment to fire cider vinegar. The angelica root honey is also an interesting flavour and provides a palatable tonic for menopausal women.

A useful honey to have around when suffering from viral or bacterial infections is garlic honey.

Garlic honey

Peel and chop or mince a whole head of garlic. Leave for at least fifteen minutes to allow the enzyme allinase to activate the allin within the garlic forming allicin. This is the powerful chemical component which helps resolve colds, coughs, sore throats, and sinus infections. Externally it can be used for skin infections. For chronic concerns, garlic helps reduce blood sugar and high blood pressure. It is said to be helpful in treating malaria and boosting immunity. It is famous as a de-wormer, should you suffer with intestinal parasites.

Place the chopped garlic in a glass jar and cover with honey, stirring with a chopstick to remove air bubbles. Leave to infuse for 3-4 weeks. The infused honey can be taken with or without the garlic pieces, depending on preference.

This honey is a useful alternative for people who cannot tolerate raw garlic.

Karen Vaughan is a qualified herbalist and acupuncturist in New York who suffers with diabetes. She shared a recipe for turmeric honey which helps to reduce inflammation and doesn't appear to affect blood sugar levels. Turmeric needs black pepper to be taken with it as an activator for all the helpful constituents.

Turmeric honey.

Take enough turmeric powder to fill a jar about two thirds full. Add 1 part freshly ground pepper and 1 part dry ginger and mix well. Then start stirring in a thin local honey (you can heat it over warm water to help thin it.) Stir in until you have a stiff paste. The precise amount varies depending upon weather and honey but the point is to put in enough to slightly cover the taste while helping the assimilation with the honey. Take a heaping teaspoonful once a day.

Honey pills and lozenges

Honey is an effective medium for delivering herbal medicine. Paul Bergner has said, "*A very active form [of taking herbs] with all the constituents is recently powdered herb decocted in hot honey. The hot honey is the consistency of water. You get as much powder into it as you can, sort of like adding flour to water to make bread dough. When the honey cools, it thickens and you get a paste. You can roll this into honey pills, roll them in licorice powder etc*".

Both Henriette Kress, the Finnish herbalist and Arizona Herbalist, Darcey Blue French, who trained with Paul Bergner, have their own methods of making honey pills.

Henriette's flu pill

This honey pill is made from six different roots plus hibiscus flowers.

- lomatium (Lomatium dissectum), anti-viral
- licorice (Glycyrrhiza glabra), soothing, anti-tussive
- echinacea (Echinacea angustifolia) immune system booster
- elecampane (Inula helenium), anti-tussive
- sweet flag (Acorus calamus), heating
- marshmallow (Althaea officinalis), soothing mucilage
- roselle (Hibiscus sabdariffa), vitamin C

The mixture started off as a herb tea mix but then she put everything into a blender, sieved it and made herbal pills by adding the resulting powder to a spruce/pine syrup she had in her fridge. Her instructions are as follows.

"For pillmaking, the moistness of the syrup + powder should be such that you can take a handful of the mix, squeeze it, and it'll show where your fingers were on the now oblong ball, which isn't wet enough to let any liquid drip off - not even one drop.

"The pills: it's easiest to make small pyramids by squeezing smidgens off that pre-squeezed ball between the tips of the thumbs and forefingers. Making hare-dropping type round pills just won't work - not after the first five or so, anyway, because this mess sticks to your hands. Drop the pills onto baking paper and, once you've formed all your pills, put the sheet into your oven at 40 C or so. You can also use a dehydrator: set that to 40 C, too. Or let things air dry, covered up to keep the flies away. NB The precise oven and the dehydrator means that your pills will be done in about 3 hours, whereas air drying means you'll have to wait for your pills for a day or two."

Darcey shared how to make honey pills with powdered herbs on the Herbwifery Forum in 2007. She described the process as *"mix the powdered herbs, and a bit of marshmallow powder (helps it to make a dough) with a bit of honey - just enough to hold it together- and work into a stiff dough, then roll into pills. These can be taken fresh, or dehydrated in the oven with the light on, or in a dehydrator to be stored on the shelf."*

Darcey used the honey pills for indigestion or nausea if she was suffering in the middle of the night, popping the pills in her mouth to let them continue their work while she returns to sleep.

We experimented with Darcey's method in a workshop in early 2017.

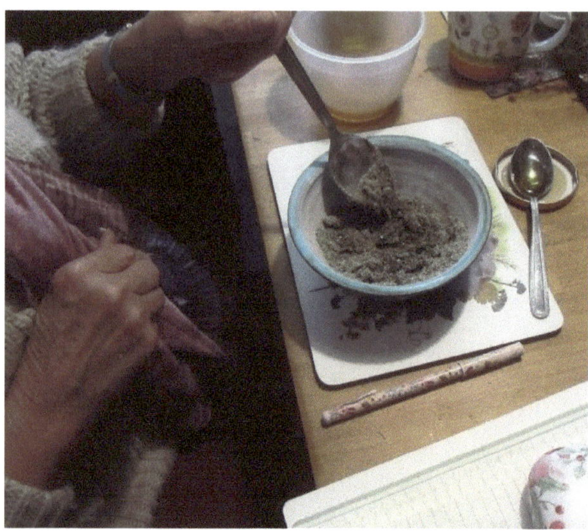

Warmed, thin honey added to freshly powdered herbs

Several different kinds of pills were made using freshly-powdered, home grown sage, thyme and elecampane root, rolled in commercially prepared marshmallow and liquorice powder.

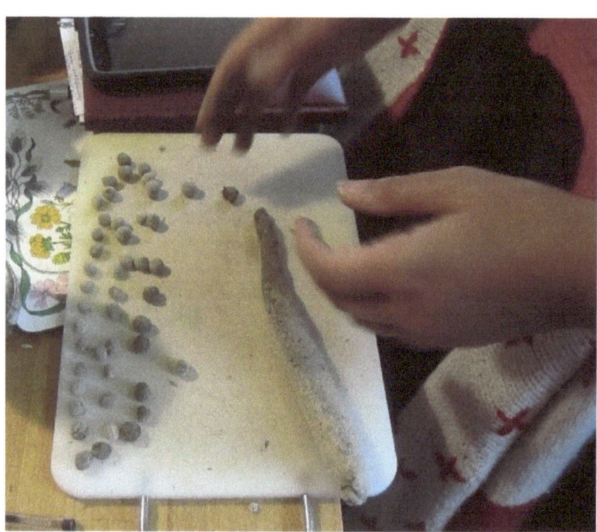

Honey/powders paste rolled into a log in marshmallow powder then pinched into pills.

In May 2009, family herbalist, Kristina Brown, wrote about making lozenges and herbal pills on the Not Dabbling in Normal blog. This is her recipe for sore throat lozenges

Herbal Lozenge Mix

3 tbsp powdered slippery elm bark
3 tbsp powdered licorice root
1 tbsp powdered echinacea root and leaf
1 tsp powdered wild cherry bark

Mix the powders together and then add enough honey to make a thick, gooey mass. It takes less honey than you'd think so start out slowly with the honey. Next add essential oils such as thyme, orange or rosemary, about 5-10 drops. When using essential oils always make sure they are safe for internal consumption as some can be quite strong. Roll the mass in more powdered slippery elm to coat and then roll out until about 1/4″ thick. Cut the dough into quarter sized pieces, roll them into a ball and place on a cookie sheet, flattening them. As you are doing this, dip them in more slippery elm if needed. Set out to dry for about 12 hours. Store in an airtight jar.

Darcey's throat lozenges

Mix slippery elm, myrrh, sage, and liquorice. She thinks this combination benefits from a drop of peppermint essential oil in the dough.

Kristina's headache pills

Mix skullcap, valerian, wood betony, chamomile and lemon balm.

Pills can be flavoured with cocoa powder or carob or herbal fruits such as rosehip or elderberry. Such flavours could be obtained by using an already infused honey rather than adding extra ingredients to the mix.

Electuaries

Electuaries are medicines made with honey or jam, sometimes made into a paste first. Ancient healers, such as Avicenna and Galen, used honey as a medium for delivering potentially unpalatable herbs. The electuaries could be very complex mixtures. Galen's *Theriac electuary* was made from a combination of sixty-four ingredients while the ancient Ayuvedic tonic, *Chyawanprash*, contains up to eighty.

Here are two different electuary recipes from Kiva Rose Hardin.

Winter Cherry Nourishing Electuary
2 parts Ashwagandha
1/2 part Nettle Seed
1 part Tulsi (Holy Basil)
2 parts Elm

This makes a lovely moistening adrenal tonic very helpful in times of stress or depletion, providing energy while relaxing the nervous system and body. It's fairly temperature neutral, and generally gentle enough for anyone.

Wild Rose Electuary
1 part Rose (petals)
1/2 part Sage (leaves)
2 parts Mallow (leaves)

She uses this combination for soothing throats and calming down belly stagnation and heat. Powdered Evening Primrose flowers can also be added as they provide extra mucilage and are helpful with digestive issues due to stress.

An electuary is made by placing your powdered herbs in a glass jar then adding heated honey slowly into the mix, stirring well. Only small amounts of honey should be added at a time so the powders don't explode and disappear! An electuary can be used immediately, but it is preferable to let them mature for a couple of weeks.

In the dark of winter, it is good to consider a warming electuary made from powdered spices mixed into honey and cooked slowly for a long time. Below is recipe from Susan Hess, who provides herbal products and workshops from her Farm at Coventry in Pottsdown, Pennsylvania.

Spiced Electuary
1/2 tsp red pepper flakes,
1 tsp whole cloves,
2 tsp coriander seeds,
2 tsp dried ginger root,
2 tsp whole black peppercorns,
2 tsp fennel seeds,
2 tsp nutmeg powder,
3 tsp cardamom seeds,
3 tsp whole allspice berries,
3 whole star anise,
3 tblsps cinnamon chips
Grind all spices together in a mortar and pestle (or electric coffee grinder if you have one) until quite finely powdered. Stir into 2 cups of honey and simmer together over the lowest heat possible double boiler for at least a day, preferably longer, but stirring often. Strain warm honey through a medium fine sieve. This will assure that you remove all the tooth-breaking hard parts, but still allow the powered bits to pass through. The finished electuary should be rich, dark and nearly paste-like in consistency. Store in a clean jar and cap tightly.

Like honey pills, electuaries can be produced for all kinds of conditions. They can be especially useful for delivering herbal combinations to children who might otherwise refuse them. Ananda Wilson, a herbalist from Northampton, Massachusetts, developed this recipe for a longevity electuary in the summer. It is based on Ayurveda principles.

Longevity Electuary
In an 8 oz jar, add:
3 tsp Ashwagandha and or Shatawari powder
3 tsp Spirulina powder
3 tsp Slippery Elm or Mallow powder
2 tsp Siberian Ginseng (Eluthero) powder
1 tsp Cardamom powder
1/2 tsp Turmeric powder
Cover almost full with good local, raw honey
Add 1 tsp of Rose hydrosol or Rose elixir. Dried Elderberry powder is optional as well.
Slowly, to avoid the infamous "cloud poof", stir with a spoon until all the powders are smoothed into the honey. Label and store. Refrigeration isn't necessary.

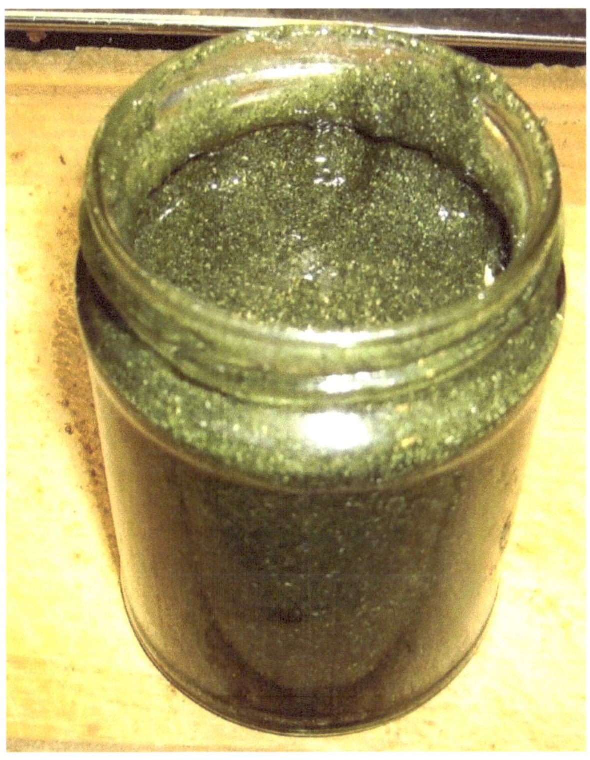

Longevity electuary

The longevity electuary is intended to be used daily, eaten by the spoonful, used on toast, stirred in warm milk with ghee, or in yogurt or smoothies. Ananda said, *"These herbs will provide you with stamina, clarity, physical and mental energy, good digestion, and strong mucous membranes. It is also a notorious aphrodisiac."*

Oxymels

The combination of infused cider vinegar and honey is often known as an oxymel or occasionally a honeygar. The practice originated in the Middle East and was brought to England following the Crusades when the medicines of Avicenna were widely used. Knights and their ladies would be offered hot oxymels when they broke their fast as a stimulating way to start the day. The standard oxymel is 2tsps cider vinegar to 2tsps of honey in a mug of boiling water.

Useful combinations

- Sage cider vinegar with rosehip honey for sore throats
- Fire cider vinegar with rosehip, plain or horseradish honey for colds/coughs/viruses
- Mint cider vinegar with mint honey (Sekanjarbin) cooling
- Mugwort cider vinegar with red clover honey for minerals

Elixirs

Honey can also be combined with brandy to provide my favourite herbal medium, an elixir. The elixir is basically a honeyed tincture made with brandy which is becoming increasingly popular amongst herbalists.

Kiva Rose Hardin has long been an advocate of elixirs because

- The sweet taste brings out the aromatic flavours and heart-healing properties of many herbs.
- Honey adds to herbal preservation and increases the shelf-life of the tincture.
- Unlike most sweet medicines, it can be used in very small doses, thanks to the particular combination of honey and alcohol. This keeps it from having much of a blood sugar impact.
- It helps to bring out the flavour and aroma of many herbs, the herb's nervine effects are enhanced, often in a significant way.
- They're extremely simple and intuitive to make

Making elixirs is fun. Whereas with tinctures, you always make single herb extractions and then combine the extracts; with elixirs, you gather a variety of herbs and combine them all with equal parts of honey and brandy. The dose is 15 drops or 1/2tsp/30 drops every 2-3 hours.

Elderberry Elixir (based on Kiva Rose's recipe)
2 Pint Jar
1/2 ounce (14g) of dried elderberries (2oz/57g fresh approx. to fill half the jar)
1 cinnamon stick,
1oz/28g root ginger peeled, sliced and chopped
Large handful of fresh or dried rosehips

Chopped peel of half a large orange
approx. 1 pint (568 ml) brandy
½-1lb (454g) honey
Place the herbs in the jar, cover with honey and mix well. Add brandy until the jar is full and mix well again. Leave to macerate for 4-6 weeks.

I have created several different elixirs. My current cough elixir has been developed further and is the only thing which helps my husband's frequent coughs.

Respiratory: flowering thyme, purple sage leaves and fennel
Uplifting: St Johns wort flowers, rose petals, lemon balm leaves, violet leaves, alpine strawberry leaves, heartease aerial parts.
Fever: red bergamot leaves and flowers, calendula flowers, flowering thyme
Colds/coughs: peppermint, flowering thyme, sage leaves (purple & green), yarrow leaves, rose petals, self-heal.
Digestive: fennel seeds and ginger root
Cough: fresh purple sage and thyme leaves (equal amount), up to three white horehound sprigs, a handful of dried elecampane root.
SAD (Seasonal Affective Disorder): Equal amounts of St John's wort flowers with lemon balm leaves

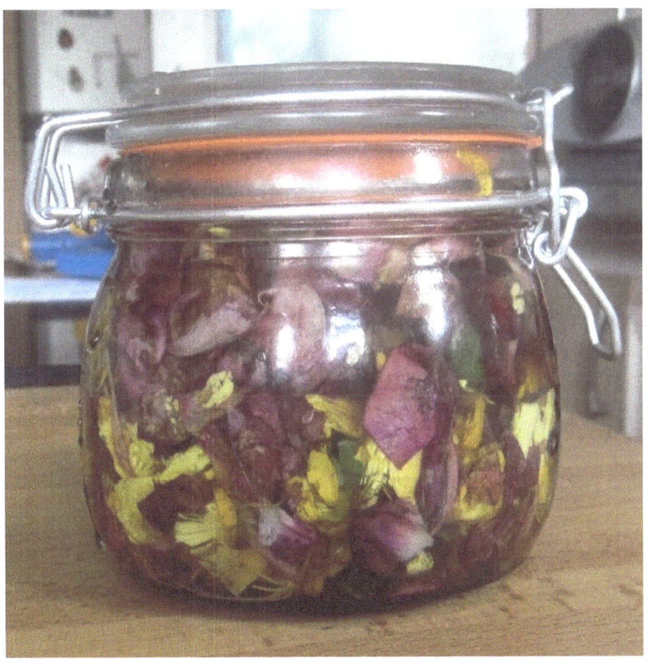

Uplifting elixir

Honey is a very special product. Whether used as a sweetening agent or medium to extract herbal properties, it offers an opportunity to nourish our bodies and bring a smile to our faces. It encourages us to be creative and enjoy our medicines and tonics. Life without honey would be an infinitely poorer place.

Notes

Chapter Six

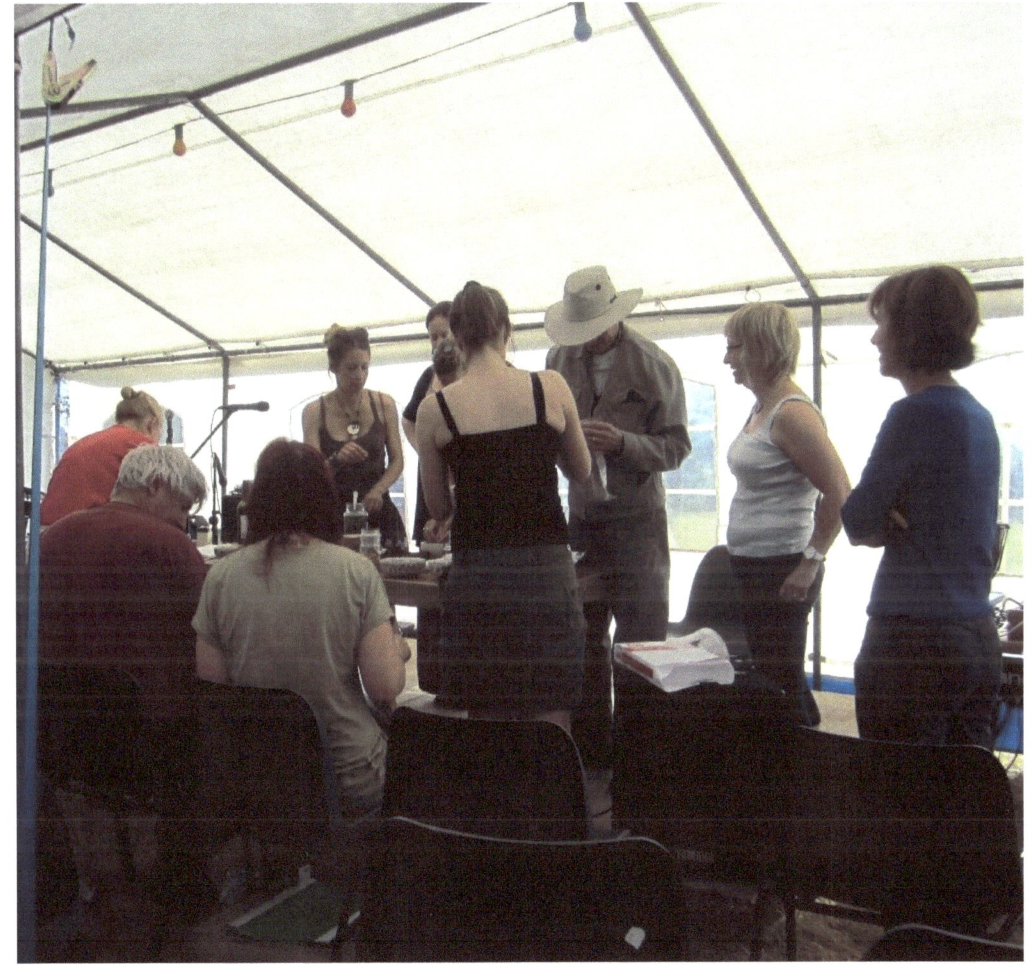

Making tonic wines at the 2012 Celebrating herbs festival

Using wine

Wine has been used as a medium for taking herbal medicines since classical times. In times when water purity could not be trusted, fermented grape juice or beers were the medium of choice. Today, that legacy is remembered in the use of tonic wines.

White wine is predominantly used for relaxing remedies and red wine works best with herbs for the digestive system. Remember that herbs can work on many different systems, so chamomile might be included in both a digestive and a stress mixture. Vervain can be used for adrenal support in a stress remedy but is also a bitter. Peppermint is best used in white wine although it is a digestive. It doesn't blend well in red wine.

It is best to use dried herbs when making a tonic wine rather than fresh to minimise the water content. The medicine can be produced in the wine bottle by removing a glassful from the bottle before adding the herbs, or in a jam jar or Kilner jar if that is easier. The wine should be left to infuse for two weeks before straining and drinking. The daily dose is 20-40mls or the equivalent of a small sherry glass. It should be sipped slowly and savoured. Medicinal wines should be used within one month.

Herbal combinations

Stress: skullcap, vervain, jasmine and wood betony
Sleep: passionflower (leaves and flowering tops), lemon balm
Digestive: crushed fennel seed, ground ivy, chamomile
Anaemia: young nettle tops, organic apricots, diced orange peel in red wine
Post surgery for broken bones: nettles, plantain (any *plantago* species, not bananas), prunes or figs, dandelion or milk thistle seeds

Historical tonics tend to favour fortified wines as well as red wines and combine several herbs and spices within the mix.

Here are four different recipes for a tonic wine.

Aromatic Wine
2-pints red wine
1/2 Tbsp sage leaves
2 Tbsps thyme leaves
2 Tbsps hyssop leaves
2 Tbsps spearmint leaves
2 Tbsps wormwood leaves
2 Tbsps marjoram herb
Use dried herbs
Chop the herbs into a coarse powder. Moisten the powders with some of the claret. Pack into a coffee machine, using parchment paper on the bottom. Pour the claret over the herbs. It should yield about 1 pint of filtered liquid.

This French formula possesses strong tonic and aromatic properties. It is useful for invalids with feeble digestions and will also help with flatulence and other digestive disturbances. Use one tablespoon at a time. For ulcers, use heated as a hot (external) compress (dip a cloth into the hot liquid).

Tonic Wine
1 pint Madeira
1 sprig wormwood
1 sprig rosemary
1 small nutmeg grated
1 inch ginger root grated
1 inch crushed cinnamon bark
12 large organic raisins
Pour off about an ounce of the wine. Place herbs in the wine. Cork the bottle tightly. Place the bottle in a dark, cool place for a week or two. Strain off the herbs.

Juliette de Bairacli' Levy's medicated wine
Several sprigs of rosemary and wormwood
6 candied cherries
2 nutmegs
1 inch cinnamon bark
Candied angelica
Bruised ginger root
1 doz large raisins
Pour over wine and leave in warm place for 1-2 weeks

Sarah's medicated wine
6-8 sprigs rosemary (fresh)
2 sprigs mugwort (dried, but can use fresh)
2 handfuls of organic apricots
2 grated nutmegs
1 inch grated ginger root
1 quill cinnamon bark broken into pieces
Place ingredients in a 2lb glass jar, cover with Madeira wine, seal with screw top lid, label and date. Leave in a warm, dark cupboard/airing cupboard for 2-4 weeks. Strain and bottle. Take one small shot glass full as required.

Christopher Hedley's iron tonic
Soak equal amounts of fresh nettle tops and organic apricots in good red wine, with a little bitter orange peel added. Soak for two weeks, strain and store in a cool place, Dose 1 or 2 dessertspoons twice daily.

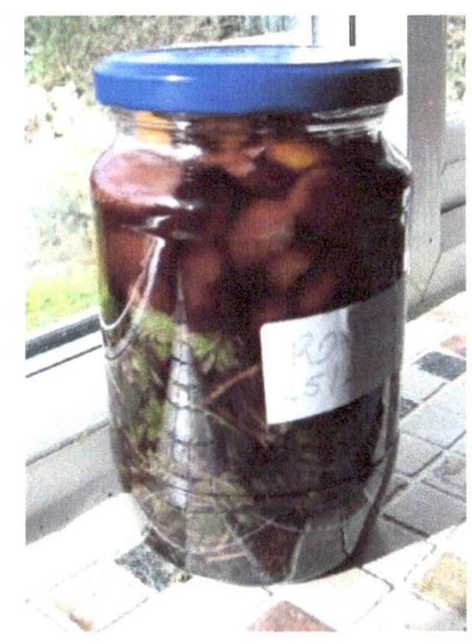

Iron tonic macerating in the windowsill

Customising tonics

To make a truly effective tonic you need to know what the recipient actually needs and what constitutional type they are. It may be you are looking to support their digestion or a particular organ in their body or an overall effect of damaging emotions such as grief.

Here is an example of making a tonic for an individual looking at their immediate needs

Karen was involved in a serious car accident which broke her pelvis and her leg in several places. The tonic made for her was based on Chris Hedley's iron tonic but with a liver component to counteract all the medication she'd been on (dandelion, burdock or milk thistle), something for the digestive system to help it start working again after all the opiate painkillers she'd taken (prunes, figs, mallow or plantain seeds) plus rose petals and rescue remedy to counteract any hospital acquired depression and generally address her emotional state. She drank the tonic whilst she was in rehabilitation and when she was discharged home. The hospital staff were delighted with how quickly she healed and her ability to walk. She returned to work within six months and is walking normally.

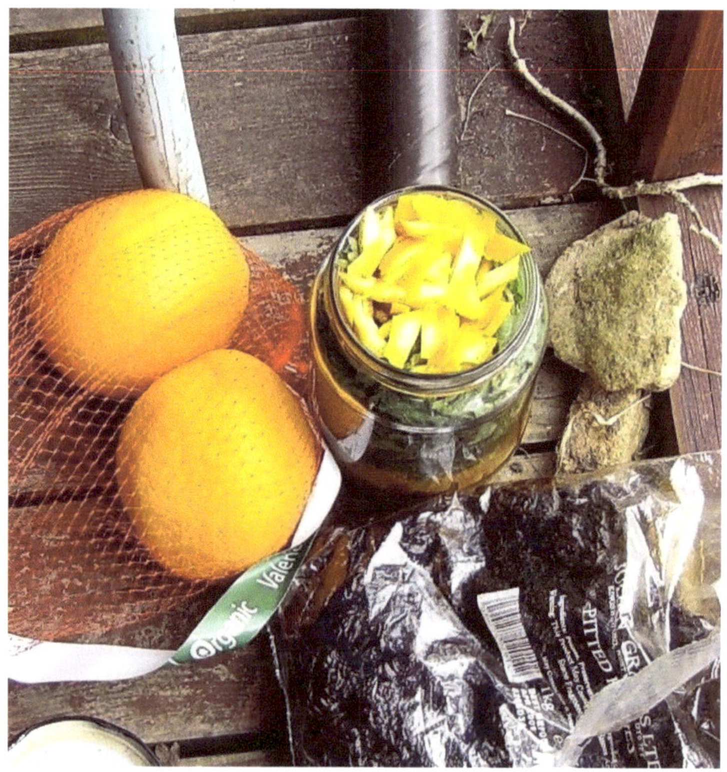

Iron tonic prepared on the summerhouse verandah

References and Further Reading

Andrews, M **The Private Tomb of Yuya and Tjuyu in the Valley of the Kings**
http://www.touregypt.net/featurestories/yuyat.htm

Bartram, T Bartram's Encyclopedia of Herbal Medicine 1998 Robinson Publication Ltd ISBN 9781854875860

Brown, D The RHS Encyclopedia of Herbs and their uses 1995 Dorling Kindersley ISBN 0 7513 0203 1

Brown, K **Family Medicine Chest: Herbal pills and lozenges**
http://notdabblinginnormal.wordpress.com/2009/05/28/family-medicine-chest-herbal-lozenges-and-pills/

Bruton-Seal, J & Seal, M Hedgerow Medicine: Harvest & make your own herbal remedies 2008 Merlin Unwin Books Ltd ISBN 978 1 873674 99 4

Buhner, SH Vital Man : Natural Health Care for men at Midlife 2003 Avery ISBN 1 58333 136 0

Church C&S **Syrups and other sweet preparations**
http://theherbarium.wordpress.com/2009/12/03/syrups-other-sweet-preparations/

Cory Su **Sweet Medicine: Making Garlic honey**
http://aquarianbath.blogspot.com/2009/07/sweet-medicine-making-garlic-honey_31.html

Edwards, G F Opening Our Wild hearts to the Healing Herbs 2000 Ash Tree Publishing ISBN 1-888123 01 X plus private correspondence

French, D B **Herbal honey pills and nothing in general**
http://desertmedicinewoman.blogspot.com/2007/09/blog-post-about-nothing-in-general.html

Green, J The Herbal Medicine-Maker's Handbook Crossing Press ISBN-13 978 0 89594 990 5

Griggs, B The Greenwitch: A Modern Women's Herbal 1993 Random House Publishing Ltd ISBN 0 09 182681 0

Hardin, K R http://bearmedicineherbals.com

Hawes, Z Wild Drugs: A Forager's guide to healing plants 2010 Octopus Publishing Group ISBN 9781856753104

Hess, S **Entertaining the electuary**
http://farmatcoventry.blogspot.com/2009/07/entertaining-electuary.html

Hoffman, D The Complete Illustrated Holistic Herbal 1996 Element Books

Kress, H http://www.henriettesherbal.com/blog/syrup-flu-pills.html

Macdonald, J http://www.herbcraft.org plus Facebook discussions

McIntyre, A The Complete Herbal Tutor 2010 Gaia Books Ltd ISBN 9781856753180

McGarry, G Brighid's Healing:Ireland's Celtic Medicine Traditions 2005 Green Magic ISBN: 0954723023

Shaw, N & Hedley, C **Herbal Remedies** 1996 Parragon Books Services Ltd ISBN 1-84164-054-9

Stapley, C Herbcraft Naturally 1994 Heartsease Books ISBN 0 9522336 1 4

Tierra, L A Kid's Herb Book for children of all ages 2000 Robert D Reed Publishers ISBN 8850003 36 6 51995

Vaughan, K **Sweet Turmeric** http://www.acupuncturebrooklyn.com/herbs/turmeric-sweet-turmeric/comment-page-1#comment-285

Wardwell, J The Herbal Home Remedy Book 1998 Versa Press ISBN-13 978 1 58017 016 1

Warner, L https://whisperingearth.co.uk/2011/12/07/how-to-make-creams-part-ii-without-emulsifiers/

Weed, S New Menopausal Years The Wise Woman Way 2002 Ash Tree Publishing ISBN 1 888123 03 6

Wilson, A **Longevity Electuary** http://plantjourneys.blogspot.com/2009/08/longevity-electuary-east-west.html

Wood, M The Practice of Traditional Western Herbalism : Basic Doctrine, Energetics and Classification 2004 North Atlantic Books ISBN 9 781556 435034 51595

Recipe Index

Recipe Index Cont.

Acknowledgements

This book would not have been possible without the love and support of my family,

my apprentices, my teachers in the world-wide herbal community

and my writing companions.

Thank you

Sarah J Head

2 August 2017

www.ingramcontent.com/pod-product-compliance
Lightning Source LLC
Chambersburg PA
CBHW040045240726
48664CB00004B/1075